*The Yellow Emperor's Classic
of Internal Medicine*

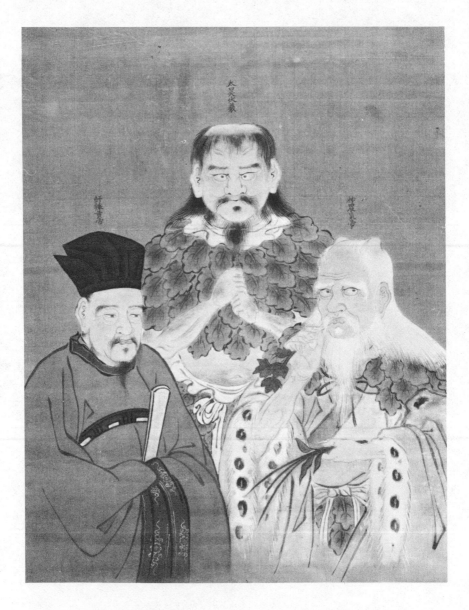

The three legendary emperors, Fu Hsi, Shen Nung, and Huang Ti, who are supposed to have founded the art of healing. From a Japanese scroll by Seibi Wake, 1798.

HUANG TI NEI CHING SU WÊN

*The Yellow Emperor's Classic
of Internal Medicine*

NEW EDITION

CHAPTERS 1–34 TRANSLATED FROM THE CHINESE
WITH AN INTRODUCTORY STUDY

BY
ILZA VEITH

UNIVERSITY OF CALIFORNIA PRESS

Berkeley, Los Angeles, London

UNIVERSITY OF CALIFORNIA PRESS
Berkeley and Los Angeles, California

UNIVERSITY OF CALIFORNIA PRESS, LTD.
London, England

© 1949 BY ILZA VEITH
FIRST UNIVERSITY OF CALIFORNIA PRESS EDITION, 1966
FIRST PAPERBACK EDITION, 1972

ISBN: 0-520-01296-8 cloth
0-520-02158-4 paper
LIBRARY OF CONGRESS CATALOG CARD NUMBER: 66-21112

Printed in the United States of America

11   12   13   14   15   16   17   18   19

FOREWORD

In most Asiatic countries modern scientific medicine has not penetrated very deeply. This is owing not only to the lack of personnel and facilities available and to the lack of a system which would enable the physician to carry out his task and to make a decent living in the rural districts where he is needed most, but also to the very foreignness of scientific medicine to the majority of the people. We cannot expect a village that lives today very much as it did centuries ago to accept modern science without far-reaching social and economic changes and without educational preparation.

As a result of these conditions most people in Asia do not receive medical care from physicians trained in modern medical schools but from indigenous practitioners who follow the precepts of ancient and medieval medicine. The medical systems of the past are still very much alive. Their study is of the greatest interest not only to the historian of medicine who wishes to understand the history of civilization but also to the modern physician whose endeavor it must be to overcome obsolete theories and practices and to replace them with the more effective techniques of scientific medicine. This however must be done gradually, in a tactful way, with a terminology and concepts familiar to the people. There can be no doubt that a thorough study of medical history will be found very helpful in such an undertaking.

In all early civilizations, moreover, medical theory had a strongly philosophical character. Hence medical books are important sources of philosophical thought and their study presents an additional key to the understanding of civilizations of the past.

China is no exception to the rule. The country has some excellent modern physicians and scientists trained in very good schools, but they are only a handful for a population of four hundred millions. The overwhelming majority of the people therefore is still served by indigenous practitioners who feel the pulse, examine the patient, reason about his symptoms, and treat him exactly as their ancestors did many centuries ago.

It is very important to know the old medical literature of China, and since the language presents considerable difficulties to the western student, texts should be translated, analyzed, and commented upon. Very few medical books have been translated so far, and those which have been were selected in a rather haphazard way. A beginning should obviously be made with the classical books that have exerted the greatest influence upon Chinese medical thought for over two thousand years. This is why every student of medical history and of Chinese culture will greatly welcome the present volume that fills a long felt gap.

The *Nei Ching*, the Classic of Internal Medicine, attributed to Huang Ti, the Yellow Emperor, is indeed a very important if not *the* most important early Chinese medical book, particularly its first part, *Su Wên*, "Familiar Conversations" between the Emperor and his physician Ch'i Pai. It is important because it develops in a lucid and attractive way a theory of man in health and disease and a theory of medicine. It does this in very much the same way as did the physicians of India who wrote the classic books of Yajurvedic medicine, or the Hippocratic physicians of Greece; that is, by using the philosophic concepts of the time and picturing man as a microcosm that reflects the macrocosm of the universe. The theory expounded in the *Nei Ching Su Wên* has remained the dominating theory of Chinese indigenous medicine to the present day.

By analyzing the contents of the book and making use of other Chinese and western sources, Dr. Ilza Veith has succeeded in giving an excellent picture of early Chinese medicine, and her translation of the *Su Wên* reads very fluently and has maintained the flavor of the original, so far as this can be done in such a version.

The interpretation of an old Chinese text is always an extraordinarily difficult task and not only for the western student. That Chinese scholars also experience great difficulties is evidenced by the fact that we know of forty-one commentaries to the *Nei Ching* written up to the end of the Ch'ing Dynasty.

If I feel privileged to say that Dr. Veith undertook this unusual task at my suggestion, it is only at once to add that the suggestion would probably never have been made nor the work undertaken, except for a precedent circumstance. And here I must pay tribute to the memory of a very unusual man, whose vision and resolution gave the project its inception. This was Mr. J. W. Lindau, an organic chemist with noteworthy contributions to his credit, who became interested in China, learned the language through his own efforts and—abandoning his business to do so—set himself one of the most difficult tasks that he could have found, the translation of the entire *Nei Ching*.

With unending patience and enthusiasm he worked on it year after year and, when he died in 1942, he left a bulky manuscript behind. Here also tribute must be paid to his devoted wife, Mrs. Theresa Lindau, who felt a strong responsibility for the manuscript and spared no effort to bring it to the attention of scholars.

It was my initial hope that it might be possible to publish the Lindau manuscript after it had been checked with the original, a hope which I clung to for a considerable time. However it is obvious that the translation of so long and difficult a work, in the course of which Mr. Lindau was developing his own knowledge of the language, must have many inconsistencies, and it was found that even the most painstaking editing could not eliminate them, and the only alternative was a quite new translation. I am sure that Mr. Lindau, had he lived and been able to observe the course of events, would have reached the same conclusion.

This is no way minimizes the work that Mr. Lindau performed nor does it detract from the honor due him as a pioneer in this field of bringing to English medical letters the classic of another century, another clime, another people. The *Nei Ching* would not have been translated except for the foresight of this exceptional man, whose name will always be remembered in admiration and gratitude in connection with the early efforts to make this classic of Chinese medicine available to the western world.

HENRY E. SIGERIST, M.D., D.Litt., LL.D.
*Formerly Director of the Johns Hopkins
Institute of the History of Medicine*

Pura, Switzerland

PREFACE TO THE NEW EDITION

DURING the years in which the translation and analysis of this oldest-known document of Chinese medicine were prepared, and at the time of the subsequent publication of this work, the subject of my study seemed to be entirely esoteric. It was then, in 1949, scarcely foreseeable that the archaic therapeutic methods based upon ancient oriental concepts of universalistic philosophy and described in the *Classic* would continue to survive vigorously and to resist the impact of modern medical science. Not only did they survive, they actually experienced a major renaissance in China, their country of origin, and beyond that, their application expanded into new territories. They spread rapidly all over Europe where they had made their entrance via France, and recently they begin to gather adherents here in the United States.

The dynamic revival of traditional medicine in present-day China has two major causes. One is the general program on the part of the People's Republic of preserving its national heritage. The other is the result of a realistic assessment of prevailing medical conditions. Upon its accession to power it had become obvious to the Communist regime that the 70,000 Western-trained physicians in all of China could not possibly provide adequate medical care for a population then numbered at 650 million. To cope with this deficiency, the government decided to make use of the 500,000 practitioners of traditional medicine in the country within the framework of public health administration.

With the revival of this medical system, fostered energetically in China, and constantly gaining momentum in the West and in Russia, the subject of this book, the time-honored dialogue about health and healing, takes on actuality and definite significance in present-day thinking. Moreover, with the steadily rising interest in Far Eastern thought and its history, the *Yellow Emperor's Classic* has gradually transcended the confines of medical history. It has in fact become a landmark in the history of Chinese civilization and even in that of other nations in the Far East, such as Japan and Tibet, in whose traditional medical systems many traces of the Chinese Classic can be detected.

The essence of medical endeavor at all times and all over the world has been the prevention and the cure of diseases and the prolongation of life. It is therefore hardly surprising that the *Yellow Emperor's Classic* should contain passages which run parallel to the modern wish to bring the acquisition of medical knowledge to the benefit of all mankind. For example, increased longevity was envisaged by the Yellow Emperor and discussed in the very opening sentence of his conversation with his minister.

Owing probably to the interest evoked by these factors, a growing demand for the *Nei Ching* required this new edition after the original publication had been exhausted. Therefore, with great pleasure I am following the invitation of the University of California Press in offering this new and revised version of my book.

I acknowledge with gratitude the constant encouragement and interest of Dr. J. B. deC. M. Saunders, Chancellor of the University of California, San Francisco Medical Center; the many helpful suggestions of Dr. Franz Michael, Professor at the Sino-Soviet Institute, George Washington University at Washington, D.C.; Hsaio-li Lindsay, also of Washington, D.C.; and the untiring assistance of my husband, Dr. Hans von Valentini Veith.

ILZA VEITH

Tiburon, California
Summer, 1965

PREFACE

ALTHOUGH some short passages of the *Nei Ching* have hitherto been translated into Western languages,[1] and brief descriptions of its contents have appeared in various textbooks on Chinese medicine, no major part of it has ever before appeared in any Western language. Yet the book constitutes the basis of Chinese and Japanese orthodox medicine. In China it is regarded as the most influential medical work in existence and has therefore been accorded first place among the medical works included in the *Ssu-k'u Ch'üan-shu*, a collection of the most important works in Chinese literature, published in 1772 under the sponsorship of the Chinese government. The contents of this book accordingly should be available to the occidental world. To make this possible Professor Sigerist communicated with the Rockefeller Foundation in order to secure a grant which would enable me to undertake the translation. In February, 1945, the Rockefeller Foundation generously bestowed upon me a fellowship for this purpose, and approved the conversion of this translation into a doctoral dissertation to be written at the Institute of the History of Medicine of the Johns Hopkins University. The fellowship was renewed the following year.

The *Huang Ti Nei Ching Su Wên* is tremendous in scope and size. It consists of about forty-four thousand ideographs, amounting, since Chinese is a very concise language, to about one hundred and twenty thousand words in translation. In addition, it was necessary to study and translate many of the numerous glosses on the text. The task of translating this work was aggravated by the absence of any adequate dictionary treating of the Chinese technical, medical and philosophical terms employed in it, and it therefore became necessary for me to develop for my own use such a dictionary from the sentences and glosses in the book.

[1] In addition to brief quotations I have found translations of short passages of the *Nei Ching* in the following works: Alfred Forke, *The World-Conception of the Chinese,* their astronomical, cosmological, and physical-philosophical speculations (London, 1925), pp. 250–252; K. Chimin Wong and Wu Lien-teh, *History of Chinese Medicine* (Tientsin, [1934]), p. 20; Percy M. Dawson, "Su-wen, the Basis of Chinese Medicine," *Annals of Medical History* VII (1925), 59–64; William R. Morse, *Chinese Medicine* (Clio Medica, XI, New York, 1934), p. 75; Franz Hübotter, *Die Chinesische Medizin zu Beginn des XX. Jahrhunderts und ihr Historischer Entwicklungsgang* (China Bibliothek der 'Asia Major', Bd. 1, Leipzig, 1929), pp. 69–71.

The translation of early Chinese texts is almost always complicated by the fact that printed editions are based upon manuscripts
which had previously gone through the hands of numerous copyists.
These copyists introduced mistakes, inserted corrupted or false
characters or left out characters or even sentences.   Such mistakes
were particularly frequent in works of the type of this medical classic,
where the meaning of the text was obscure and beyond the compre-
hension of the copyists, who frequently were mere clerks rather than
scholars.   Thus it was necessary, whenever there was a possibility
of a mistake or an omission, to study analogous sentences and to
consider the possibility of using characters from these analogous
sentences to clear up the difficulties.   Fortunately, however, Chinese
classical texts are given to a great deal of parallelism in contents and
sentence structure, so that in many cases obscure points could be
elucidated.[2]

But even where sporadic difficulties, such as mistakes and omis-
sions, do not exist, classical Chinese constantly presents a great number of problems.   Punctuation is completely unknown and there
is no indication whatsoever as to where one sentence ends and the
next one begins.   The rhythm of the text must supply the function
of periods, commas, colons, etc., making great difficulties for the
reader.   In modern Chinese writing, as it was introduced through the
"literary renaissance" movement of Dr. Hu Shih, the classical form
has been abandoned and replaced by the spoken language, which is
better suited for scientific exactness than were the philosophically
shaded meanings of classical expressions.   The classical Chinese
scholar, however, took pride in expressing highly complicated sentences with as few characters as possible.   In such cases, as in the
Nei Ching, even the smallest grammatical aids are lacking and the
translator or even the Chinese reader is frequently confronted by
Pythian oracles.

The well-known sinologist Wilhelm Grube states this problem
when he writes that "it is by no means unusual that one and the

[2] For a particularly striking example of parallelism in contents and sentence structure,
see chapter 22 of the translation.   In this chapter, which deals with a system of prognosis,
every paragraph describing the course of the disease during the year is repeated verbatim,
except where two sets of designations for the seasons are employed.   Another example may
be found in chapter 19, where the process of aging is described five times in almost identical
words.   If in such cases the text contained characters which obviously did not fit into the
context and were clearly the result of an error of the copyist, the paragraphs with the identical
contents furnished the solution for the translation of the doubtful ideograph.

same Chinese sentence admits [many] grammatically different interpretations.''[3] Dr. Erich Hackmann quotes an example that illus-
trates Dr. Grube's words by means of the following sentence: *Ming
lai yeh ch'ü* (明 來 夜 去). These four characters represent the
following concepts: 1. *ming*: light, to be light; 2. *lai*: to come; 3. *yeh*:
night; 4. *ch'ü*: to leave. The simplest way of combining these four
concepts is: "Light (the day) comes, the night departs." But the
sentence can also mean: "If the day arrives, the night departs," or
"When the day arrived, the night departed," or it can even mean:
"He (she, it, they) arrived during the day and he (she, it, they)
left at night."[4] These are comparatively simple variations of one
sentence. But it stands to reason that in a more complicated context, especially if the sentence has an abstract and philosophical
significance, the possible variations can change the meaning of the
sentence to a large degree.

Another factor that renders translation difficult is the fact that
one character can have an infinite variety of meanings, sometimes
of the exactly opposite nature. Some of those taken at random
from a dictionary are 逆 *ni*: "to disobey, to rebel, to oppose; refractory, contrary, rebellious; to meet, to accord with, to anticipate."
Or 蒙 *mêng*: "to cover, to conceal; dull, stupid; an untaught child;
to receive from a superior; depreciatory term, I, my, to meet with,
to leave; to cheat, etc." In spoken Chinese the various meanings
are frequently indicated by the combination of the character with
another one of approximately the same meaning. In classical texts,
however, the character stands by itself, and its particular meaning
in each individual case must be chosen according to the context and
analogy.

Any translation that has to confront all the difficulties mentioned
above can proceed only at a very slow and careful pace. Very little
has been translated from the Chinese that has not—at least in part—
been criticized by other sinologists who read different meanings into
individual sentences. Philologists, as a rule, employ Chinese aid,
and all the outstanding translations of Chinese works, such as
James Legge's translation, *The Chinese Classics*,[5] and Édouard

---

[3] P. Hinneberg, *Die Kultur der Gegenwart* (Berlin, 1913), I, pt. 5, p. 61.

[4] Heinrich Hackmann, *Chinesische Philosophie* (Geschichte der Philosophie in Einzeldar-
stellungen, Bd. 5, München, 1927), p. 18.

[5] J. Legge, *The Chinese Classics*, with a translation, critical and exegetical notes, prolegomena and copious indexes (5 vols. in 8 pts., Oxford, 1893-1895).

Chavannes' *Les Mémoires historiques de Se-ma Ts'ien*,[6] were made
with the assistance of Chinese collaborators. But even in collaboration with a Chinese—and it is not easy to find among the modern
Chinese college students in this country persons who are sufficiently
acquainted with ancient Chinese literature and philosophy and
have received the old style literary training—a careful philological
study of a work of the size of the *Nei Ching* would take several
decades.

Yet for the purpose of making this book available to the occidental
medical historian it seems less urgent to study each character and
sentence in its philological derivation than to bring out the actual
contents of the work. Professor Homer H. Dubs, the translator of
Pan Ku's History of the Former Han Dynasty,[7] whom I consulted
at the beginning of my work, advised me to make a rough translation
of the *Nei Ching*; by means of such a translation it would then be
possible to find passages which warrant more detailed and careful
translation. In accepting Dr. Dubs' advice I have also followed
the example of Dr. Sigerist, who stated in his preface to his *Studien
und Texte zur Frühmittelalterlichen Rezeptliteratur*:[8] "For the moment,
the main point is not to publish critical editions based on philological analysis before we have some concept of the nature of the material, before we know what is of value, what is worthless, and what
bearing it may have."

It should be realized, therefore, that the translation of this classic
represents the approach of a medical historian rather than that of a
Chinese philologist. It is hoped that this preliminary study will
serve as a starting point for further work on the text, with more
specific attention to its many linguistic problems.

In the course of its existence the *Nei Ching* has been annotated,
rearranged, and supplemented many times. There are a great
number of repetitions; sometimes entire chapters are repeated with
only minor changes of rewording. Although it is my intention to
translate the entire work, I am convinced that the first thirty-four

[6] Se-ma-Ts'ien (Ssu-ma Ch'ien), *Les Mémoires historiques de Se-ma-Ts'ien*, traduits et
annotés par Édouard Chavannes (5 vols. in 6 pts., Paris, 1895–1905).

[7] Pan Ku, *The History of the Former Han Dynasty*, a critical translation, with annotations
by Homer H. Dubs with the collaboration of Jen T'ai and P'an Lo-chi (Baltimore, 1938).

[8] Henry E. Sigerist, *Studien und Texte zur Frühmittelalterlichen Rezeptliteratur* (Studien zur
Geschichte der Medizin, Heft 13, Leipzig, 1923), p. iv.

chapters—the part here translated—contain nearly all the basic ideas of the *Nei Ching*.

These ideas require interpretation and detailed analysis, so as to establish their place in Chinese medical and philosophical thought. The terminology and conceptual content of this thought are in general as symbolic and abstract as those found in Chinese religious works, making doubly difficult the task of the translator, and imposing a burden of interpretation on both the analyst and the reader. The analysis that follows should help the reader understand those parts of the translation where it was not possible to avoid the abstractions of the text.

It is hoped that the illustrations will aid in this process. Most of them were taken from the oriental collection of Dr. Howard A. Kelly, which is deposited in the Institute of the History of Medicine, at the Johns Hopkins University. The books of the Kelly collection, although of a more recent date than the *Nei Ching*, are largely based upon this classic, and their illustrations depict medical theories which are similar to those expressed in the *Nei Ching* itself.

ILZA VEITH

ACKNOWLEDGMENTS

In the preparation of this work I have availed myself of the help and kindness of many institutions and individuals. In particular, I owe an immense debt of gratitude to Professor Henry E. Sigerist, without whose guidance and inspiration this task could not have been undertaken and carried out.

I also wish to acknowledge my indebtedness to the other members of the Institute of the History of Medicine of the Johns Hopkins University. Dr. Edward H. Hume has been generous in reading and making helpful criticism of both my translation and analysis. I have also received constructive advice from Professor Homer H. Dubs, formerly of Columbia University, from Dr. Karl August Wittfogel, also of Columbia University, and from Dr. Shih Yu-chung, of the Far Eastern Department of the University of Washington. Dr. Kemp Malone, Chairman of the Department of English, the Johns Hopkins University, has been most encouraging in his interest. Dr. Arthur W. Hummel of the Division of Orientalia, Library of Congress, has been most helpful with suggestions and materials. Finally, I wish to acknowledge the courtesy of the librarians at the Johns Hopkins University.

ILZA VEITH

TABLE OF CONTENTS

Introduction: Analysis of the *Huang Ti Nei Ching Su Wên*   1

Examination of its Age and Authorship   4

The Philosophical Foundations   9

    Tao   10

    The Theory of Tao Applied to the *Nei Ching*   12

    Yin and Yang   13

    The Theory of Yin and Yang Applied to the *Nei Ching*   15

    The Five Elements and the System of Numbers   18

    The Celestial Stems   24

Anatomical and Physiological Concepts   25

Diagnosis   42

Diseases of the *Nei Ching*   49

Therapeutic Concepts   53

Acupuncture and Moxibustion   58

Appendix I: Chapter 103 of the *Ssu-k'u Ch'üan-shu*   77

Appendix II: Preface of the Commentator Wang Ping (762 A.D.)   81

Appendix III: Preface of Kao Pao-hêng and Lin I (1078 A.D.)   87

Bibliography   91

Translation of the *Nei Ching*: Chapters 1–34   95

LIST OF ILLUSTRATIONS

1. The Kidneys.................................... 26
2. The Three Burning Spaces....................... 27
3. The Liver..................................... 29
4. The Gall Bladder.............................. 31
5. The Large Intestines........................... 32
6. The Small Intestines........................... 33
7. The Pericardium............................... 35
8. The Heart.................................... 36
9. The Bladder................................... 37
10. Position of the Five Viscera.................... 38
11. The Stomach................................. 39
12. The Spleen................................... 40
13. The Internal Organs.......................... 41
14. The Three Pulses............................. 44
15. Methods of Palpation......................... 46
16. Diagram showing the Arrangement of the Pulses of the Viscera
      and the Bowels.............................. 48
17. The Vessels of the Legs....................... 60
18. The Vessels of the Arms....................... 61
19. The Kidney Vessel and the Heart Vessel........ 63
20. The "Sunlight" Vessels........................ 64
21. Acupuncture Chart............................ 66
22. Acupuncture Needles.......................... 67
23. Acupuncture Needle Case, and Needles.......... 69
24. Moxibustion Chart............................ 71

INTRODUCTION

Analysis of the *Huang Ti Nei Ching Su Wên*

W ESTERN medicine reached China in the early 17th century, when the Jesuit fathers who had been trained in medicine[1] and the physicians employed by the East India Companies[2] began to extend their activities to Chinese patients. The first organized effort to introduce Western medicine into China was made upon the realization by the American Board of Commissioners for Foreign Missions that medicine could serve as an aid in the spreading of Christianity.[3] Following the inauguration of the Medical Missionary Society in China in 1838,[4] the scope of activity of Western medicine increased rapidly, and in the last third of the 19th century a considerable number of Chinese cities had well-run hospitals of fair size. The same impetus contributed to the founding of several small medical schools, some of which, during the 20th century, grew to impressive proportions.

In the twenties and thirties of this century it became a generally accepted fact among the population of China that these medical schools were teaching Western medicine; the hospitals were dispensing Western medicine, and the individual physicians were treating their patients with Western methods. This does not mean that the orthodox Chinese physician has now disappeared, or that he has become impoverished for lack of patients. On the contrary, he has held his own, not only in the outlying regions where Western medicine is unobtainable, but even in the large cities where a great many Chinese visit their own traditional doctors by their own choice; not necessarily because they cannot afford to pay for the services of

---

1. J. P. Du Halde, "The Art of Medicine among the Chinese," in *A Description of the Empire of China* (2 vols., n.p., 1738), II, 183–214.
2. H. B. Morse, *The Chronicles of the East India Company Trading to China, 1635–1843* (Oxford, 1929).
3. W. Lockhart, *The Medical Missionary in China* (n.p., 1861).
4. "The Medical Missionary Society in China," Address with Minutes of Proceedings (Canton, 1838), and K. S. Latourette, *A Century of Protestant Missions in China* (Shanghai, 1907), pp. 175 ff.

Western physicians—who as a matter of fact often charge less than their Chinese colleagues—and not necessarily because the number of Western trained physicians is too small to take care of additional patients, but for the simple reason that they have greater confidence in those physicians who have received their training according to ancient patterns.[5]

The tendency to adhere to tradition, however, is not by itself sufficient to determine the selection of doctors; nor would religious superstitions and prejudice against foreign methods carry weight against superior practices. The confidence in the Chinese orthodox doctor is kept alive by the fact that Chinese medicine is known to have brought about enough successful cures to take from it the stigma of hazard.[6] In his analysis of the nature of Chinese medicine Dr. T. Nakayama writes: "Is it possible to consider ancient Chinese medicine as a real science? This is a troublesome question. To the moderns, indeed, there seems nothing scientific about it. On the contrary, it is covered with a prehistoric mystic patina, and sometimes appears to be scarcely comprehensible. Nevertheless, when one is aware of its great therapeutic efficacity, one cannot deny its value."[7]

This preference for orthodox Chinese physicians is especially noticeable when treatment for internal diseases is desired. The Chinese have learned to appreciate the obvious blessings of modern surgery;[8] moreover, surgery itself is almost without tradition in China and thus did not displace indigenous practices. The reason for the lack of the study of anatomy and surgery is explained by Dr. Nakayama:"Anatomy and surgical operations were unknown in Chinese medicine, for it had no need of them; it possessed the superiority of internal therapy, making unnecessary all operations and even all [knowledge of] anatomy. But this the general public did not understand."[9]

5. Oskar Eckstein, "Über altchinesische Medizin," *Schweizerische medizinische Wochenschrift*, 1925, No. 15, pp. 2–8.
6. Edward H. Hume, *Doctors East, Doctors West* (New York, 1946), p. 122; see also Eckstein, *op. cit.*, p. 2.
7. T. Nakayama, *Acupuncture et Médecine Chinoise Vérifiées au Japon*, traduites du japonais par T. Sakurazawa et G. Soulié de Morant et précédées d'une préface de G. Soulié de Morant (Paris, 1934), p. 17.
8. Hume, *Doctors*, p. 81; Eckstein, *op. cit.*, p. 2.
9. Nakayama, *Acupuncture et Médecine Chinoise*, p. 20.

Here Dr. Nakayama oversimplifies the problem. It was not entirely the superiority of Chinese internal medicine that made surgery unnecessary, but the Confucian tenets of the sacredness of the body, which counteracted any tendency toward the development of anatomical studies and the practice of surgery. Nevertheless, Chinese medical history records two eminent surgeons, Pien Ch'iao and Hua T'o. Pien Ch'iao[10] (扁 鵲) practiced in the second century B.C., and legend ascribes to him such skilful use of anesthesia that he was able to operate painlessly and even to exchange successfully the hearts of two patients. Hua T'o[11] (華 陀), whose writings on surgery and anesthesia became known around 190 A.D., is definitely established as an historical personality, famous for his excellent operative technique. Unfortunately, Hua T'o's works were destroyed; his surgical practices fell into disuse, with the exception of his method of castration, which continued to be practiced. Due to the religious stigma attached to the practice of surgery, the social

10. According to the historian Ssu-ma Ch'ien who recorded Pien Ch'iao's life history in the 105th chapter of his *Shih chi* (史 記), the physician lived in the 6th century B.C. For an annotated translation of Ssu-ma Ch'ien's biography see Franz Hübotter, "Berühmte Chinesische Aerzte des Altertums," *Archiv für Geschichte der Medizin*, Bd. VII, Heft 2 ([Leipzig, 1913]). The numerous anecdotes, however, which tell of Pien Ch'iao's achievements as a surgeon and diagnostician extend from the 5th to the 2nd century B.C. and over a great variety of places distant from each other. It is therefore believed that the name Pien Ch'iao constituted a laudatory term which was applied to many physicians in the course of four centuries. The most recent physician who was known under the name of Pien Ch'iao was Ch'in Yüeh-jen (秦 越 人), who lived about 255 B.C. and to whom is ascribed the authorship of the *Nan Ching*, or "Difficult Classic," a treatise which consists of explanations of 81 difficult passages selected from the *Nei Ching*. For further information on Pien Ch'iao see Franz Hübotter, *Die Chinesische Medizin*, pp. 12, 92; K. C. Wong and Lienteh Wu, *History of Chinese Medicine* (Tientsin, [1932?]), pp. 14–16, 28, 30, 36–37, 39, etc.; Edward H. Hume, *The Chinese Way in Medicine* (Baltimore, 1940) pp. 75–78, 173.

11. The biography of Hua T'o, who lived from about 190 to 265 A.D., is recorded in the *Annals of the Later Han Dynasty* (Hou Han Shu, Em. 72, B:5b–9a). According to this source and many other accounts, Hua T'o excelled as a surgeon and is held to have applied general anesthesia which he produced by means of a drug dissolved in wine. The ingredients of this wine, known as *ma-fei-san* (麻 沸 散), which literally translated means "bubbling drug medicine," or *ma-yao* (麻 藥) meaning in its modern translation "anesthetic," are not known. However, according to a marginal comment of the noted sinologist Dr. Erich Hauer, it seems to have been his opinion that *ma-fei* (麻 沸) means opium. For further information on Hua T'o see Franz Hübotter, "Zwei Berühmte Chinesische Ärzte des Altertums, Ch'un Yü-i und Hua T'o," *Mitteilungen der Deutschen Gesellschaft für Natur- und Völkerkunde Ostasiens*, Bd. XXI, Teil A. (Tokyo, 1925); Wong and Wu, *op. cit.*, pp. 31, 33, 35–38; Hume, *Chinese Way*, pp. 86–88, 104.

position accorded to the surgeon became increasingly lower and thus made a revival of Chinese surgery impossible.[12]

EXAMINATION OF THE AGE AND THE AUTHORSHIP OF THE NEI CHING

While there are very few texts on anatomy and surgery, the body of ancient writings on internal diseases is voluminous; and it is therefore of small wonder that physicians trained in the art of their own classical authorities appeal strongly to the Chinese with their inherent belief in the sacredness of their past.   Even many of those Chinese physicians who have received their training abroad or at modern medical schools in China have not been able to free themselves completely from their early awe of the founders of Chinese medicine.   This is exemplified by the report of Dr. E. V. Cowdry of the Anatomical Laboratory, Peking Union Medical College, who writes: "In the Office of Imperial Physicians, an image of Huangti, the mythical father of Chinese medicine, is worshipped twice a year and the practice condoned by Chinese who have taken their medical degrees in the United States and who apparently see nothing incongruous in it."[13]

Whether Huang Ti—the Yellow Lord,[14] or the Yellow Emperor as this name is most frequently translated—was a mythical or an actual personality is very difficult to decide.   Modern historiography tends

12. Wang Chi-min, "China's Contribution to Medicine in the Past," *Annals of Medical History*, VIII (1926), 192–201, and Lien-teh Wu, "Past and Present Trends in the Medical History of China," *The Chinese Medical Journal*, LIII (1938), 313–322.

13. E. V. Cowdry, "Taoist Ideas of Anatomy," *Annals of Medical History*, III (1921), 309.
   This practice of paying homage to medical sages has a long tradition.   It is significant that the three main recipients of the semiannual worship were emperors whose deification was based upon their medical achievements rather than upon their merits in government. The idea for the first three-emperor-temple was conceived in 747 A.D. by the emperor T'ang Ming-huang (唐 明 皇), when he ordered the erection of a place of worship of Fu-hsi, Shen-nung, and Huang Ti.   In 1295 the emperor Yuan Ch'eng-tsung (元 成 宗) enlarged upon the idea of worship of the ancient physicians by decreeing that a three-emperor-temple be built in each district in China.   In the course of time, four ministers and ten ancient physicians were added to the three emperors and worship was held every spring and autumn according to the Confucian rites.   For additional information on medical deities see Lee T'ao, "Ten Celebrated Physicians and Their Temple," *Chinese Medical Journal*, LVIII (1940), 267–274; and Lee S. Huizenga, "Lü Tsu and His Relation to Other Medicine Gods," *ibid.*, pp. 275–283.

14. This translation of Huang Ti as "Yellow Lord" was suggested to me by Dr. Homer H. Dubs.

to relegate him to the realm of legend.[15]   Genealogies of Chinese dynasties which are generally appended to Chinese dictionaries list him as the third of China's first five rulers and ascribe to him the period of 2697–2597 B.C.[16]   Yet in spite of these precise dates, the Age of the Five Rulers which is said to have lasted for 647 years (2852–2205 B.C.) is called the "Legendary Period."[17]   Even Giles adhered to this traditional dating, and he devoted this short paragraph in his *Biographical Dictionary* to Huang Ti: "Huang Ti (黃 帝) the Yellow Emperor, one of the most famous of China's legendary rulers.   He is said to have reigned 2696–2598 B.C. and to have been miraculously conceived by his mother, Fu Pao (附 寶), who gave birth to him on the banks of the river Chi (姬) from which he took his surname.   His personal name was Yu-hsiung (有 熊), taken from that of his hereditary principality; and also Hsien-yüan (軒 懷), said by some to be the name of a village near which he dwelt, by others to refer to wheeled vehicles of which he was the inventor, as well as of armor, ships, pottery, and other useful appliances.   The close of his long reign was made glorious by the appearance of the phoenix and that mysterious animal, known as the Ch'i lin (variously identified with the unicorn and the giraffe) in token of his wise and humane administration."[18]   However, this relegation of the Yellow Emperor to prehistoric times is made in spite of the fact that Ssu-ma Ch'ien (司 馬 遷), the great historian of the second century B.C., began his *Historical Records* with an account of Huang Ti, whom he defined as the founder of Chinese civilization and the first human ruler of the empire.[19]

Yet, quite irrespective of the controversies of the historians in regard to the existence of the Yellow Emperor, his place in the hierarchy of the Chinese deities is firmly established, because to him is attributed the authorship of the *Nei Ching Su Wên*, the classic treatise on internal medicine, and supposedly the oldest medical book extant.

15. C. P. Fitzgerald, *China, A Short Cultural History* (New York, 1938), pp. 13–15; Edward T. Williams, *A Short History of China* (New York, 1928), pp. 637 ff.
16. Herbert Allen Giles, *A Chinese English Dictionary* (London, 1892), p. 1364.
17. R. H. Mathews, *A Chinese-English Dictionary* (Cambridge, Mass., 1944), p. 1165.
18. Herbert Allen Giles, *A Biographical Dictionary* (London, 1898), p. 338.
19. Chavannes, *Les Mémoires historiques de Se-ma Ts'ien.*

It is extremely difficult to determine with any degree of certainty
the actual date of composition of the *Huang Ti Nei Ching Su Wên*—
the *Yellow Emperor's Classic of Internal Medicine*—for this is obviously connected with the question referred to earlier, that of the
earthly existence of Huang Ti.   Dr. E. T. Hsieh of the Anatomical
Laboratory of the Peking Union Medical College, in his excellent
"Review of Ancient Chinese Anatomy," seems to be of the firm
opinion that the Yellow Emperor was the author of the great classic.
He attributes the invention of the art of writing to the Yellow
Emperor[20] and, after having thus created the basis which alone could
have made it possible that the text was written at such an early
time, he proceeds to indicate the fundamental importance of the
Huang Ti Nei Ching Su Wên: "The works of Huang-ti, written over
four thousand years ago, 2697 B.C., are the most interesting and
original of the great Chinese medical classics.   They stand at the
basis of Chinese native medicine."[21]   It is undoubtedly true that
the *Nei Ching Su Wên* does constitute the basis of Chinese native
medicine, but it seems highly unlikely that the Yellow Emperor was
its author.   Ssu-ma Kuang, whose attitude towards the legends of
the heroic age was uncritical and who acknowledged the earthly existence of Huang Ti,[22] nevertheless wrote in a letter to Fan Ching-
jen: "To state that Huang Ti was the real author of the *Su Wên* is
open to serious doubt.   The emperor has to attend to the affairs of
the state; how is it possible for him to sit all day long and discuss
problems of medicine with his minister Ch'i Pai? The book is written
between the Chou and Han dynasties by some one who antedates it
so as to enhance its value."[23]

20. In this he follows the traditional view rather than any historical evidence, for no traces
    of writing prior to 2000 B.C. have been found.   "Since the First World War our direct
    archeological knowledge of China before the first millenium B.C. has been carried back
    to the Chalcolithic by the discovery of painted-pottery cultures in northern China and
    to the second millenium B.C. by the excavations at An-yang in Honan.   It is still true
    that no actual written document can be dated with certainty before the twelfth century
    B.C., but the names of kings of the Shang-Yin Dynasty on the oracle bones from the site
    take us to about the middle of the second millenium.   It is hardly likely that future
    finds will carry written records back before 2000 B.C." (William F. Albright, *From the
    Stone Age to Christianity* [Baltimore, 1940], p. 5).
21. E. T. Hsieh, "A Review of Ancient Chinese Anatomy," *Anatomical Record*, XX (1921),
    98–99.   Dr. Hsieh's opinions about the origin and the nature of the *Nei Ching* are inter-
    esting, for they combine adherence to traditional historical belief with the critical attitude
    of a scientist trained in Western medicine.
22. Fitzgerald, *op. cit.*, p. 208.
23. Wong and Wu, *History of Chinese Medicine*, p. 17.

This is rather vague. It places the authorship of a work that has so profoundly influenced Chinese medical thinking within a period which covers nearly one thousand years. However, later research has been equally unable to find a definite date or author for the *Yellow Emperor's Classic on Internal Medicine*. Dr. Wang Chi-min in his brilliant summary of "China's Contribution to Medicin in the Past" said in discussing the classic: ". . . historical researches proved that this work was not composed by him [Huang Ti] but was a later production, written probably about 1000 B.C. It is the most important medical classic. What the *Four Books*[24] are to the Confucianists, the *Nei Ching* is to the native doctors. Upon it is built most of the medical literature of China and so important is it considered by medical men that even at the present time, three thousand years after it was written, it is still regarded as the greatest authority."[25]

Dr. Wang's approximation of the date of composition (1000 B.C.) has been modified by the analysis of Léon Wieger, S.J., who, upon the study of the *Su Wên*, which constitutes a substantial part of the *Nei Ching Su Wên*, concluded: "I attribute to this period (the first Han dynasty) the analysis of the *Su-Wên*, *Simple Questions*, because the style of this work does not at all permit us to place earlier the edition which has come to us, and because it certainly existed under this form at this epoch. But its contents are older. It sums up the experimental, physiological knowledge of all the centuries which preceded, for it systematized it in one chapter. . . . This chapter is certainly later than Lao-tze, beginning of the fifth century; but I estimate that its outline was prior to the end of the fourth century."[26]

In the hope that the largest and most complete Chinese bibliographical dictionary[27] might be helpful in giving more details about

24. The "Four Books" are the *Ta Hsüeh* or the *Great Study*, the *Chung Yung* or the *Invariable Mean*, the *Lun Yü* or *Miscellaneous Conversations*, and *Meng-tzu* containing the conversations of Mencius with the princes and grandees of his time; see A. Wylie, *Notes on Chinese Literature* (Shanghai, 1922).

25. Wang Chi-min, "China's Contribution to Medicine," pp. 192 ff.

26. Léon Wieger, S.J., *Histoire des Croyances religieuses et des Opinions philosophiques en Chine depuis l'Origine, jusqu'à nos Jours* (Sienhsien, Hokienfu, 1917), pp. 313-317. The quotation used here is taken from a translation by Dawson, "Su-wen, the Basis of Chinese Medicine," p. 59.

27. *Ssu-k'u ch'üan-shu tsung-mu t'i-yao* 四庫全書總目提要 [A Complete Bibliography of the Imperial Library], ed. Yung Jung and others (Shanghai, The Commercial Press, Ltd., 1933).

the origin of the medical canon, I have translated the chapter[28] which deals with the *Huang Ti Nei Ching Su Wên*. According to this chapter the earliest mention of the medical work can be found in the Annals of the Former Han Dynasty (206 B.C.–25 A.D.), where it appeared as *Huang Ti Nei Ching* and was listed as having eighteen fascicles. The treatise of *Su Wên*[29] itself was first mentioned by the great physician of the second century A.D., Chang Chung-ching,[30] who quoted it in his famous *Treatise on Typhoid Fever*. During the Chin dynasty (265–419 A.D.) the eighteen fascicles of the *Huang Ti Nei Ching* were again mentioned in the preface of a medical book by Huang-fu Mi.[31] But its full title, *Huang Ti Nei Ching Su Wên*, was recorded for the first time in the *Annals of the Sui Dynasty* (589–618 A.D.). At that time, however, ten of the eighteen previously mentioned books had disappeared, for the treatise was listed as containing only eight books.

Hence the edition of the *Huang Ti Nei Ching Su Wên*, consisting of twenty-four books—as it has come to us—owes its present form largely to its most famous commentator, Wang Ping of the Tang dynasty, who claimed to have discovered and used its original edition. In 762, after completing his commentary upon the work, he wrote a preface to it in which he stated that by combining various texts and by adding his commentary he had expanded the work into twenty-four books and sub-divided them into eighty-one chapters.[32] During the decade of 1068–1078 in the reign of Shên Tsung (神宗) of the Sung dynasty, the *Huang Ti Nei Ching Su Wên* was again commented upon and re-edited under imperial auspices. The

28. *Ibid.*, chapter 103. The translation will be found in Appendix I.

29. The two characters of Su Wên have been translated in various ways. Su (素) means: plain; white, unornamented, ordinary, simple. Wên (問) means: to ask, to inquire. According to the form of the treatise it might be translated as "Questions and Answers." Léon Wieger has translated it as "Simple Questions". Dr. Homer H. Dubs suggested "Interpretation of Problems."

30. Chang Chung-ching (張仲景) was the most famous of the three great doctors of the Han dynasty, the other two being Tsang Kung and Hua T'o. The only fact known about Chang Chung-ching's life is that he was mayor of Chang-sha around the year 195. Because of his *Treatise on Typhoid Fever* he is frequently spoken of as the Chinese Hippocrates. See Wang Chi-min, "China's Contribution to Medicine," p. 196.

31. Huang-fu Mi (皇甫謐) (215–282 A.D.) was the author of the *Chia I Ching*, which deals with acupuncture and moxa treatment. Wong and Wu, *History of Chinese Medicine*, pp. 59–60.

32. See translation of Wang Ping's preface in Appendix II.

editors, Kao Pao-hêng and Lin I, although basing much of their work upon Wang Ping's commentaries, yet felt the need for extensive rearrangement and revision of the text with the purpose of elucidating its meaning.[33]

It is obvious that any work that has undergone the fate of *The Yellow Emperor's Canon of Internal Medicine* contains but little of its authentic original text; it is also clear that its various commentators have frequently obscured rather than elucidated its meaning.[34] It seems impossible to determine now how much of the original text remains; especially since in former times it was difficult to distinguish text from commentary.[35] Nevertheless it is fair to assume that a great part of the text existed during the Han dynasty, and that much of it is of considerably older origin, possibly handed down by oral tradition from China's earliest history. The fact that some of its historical and geographical allusions, of which there are but a small number, and its literary construction refer to a time later than that of the Yellow Emperor does not necessarily prove a more recent authorship; these anachronisms may have been inserted later. On the other hand, the fact that the work is ascribed to Huang Ti and that he figures frequently in its pages, cannot serve to prove his existence, nor his connection with the authorship of the text. In China, where values are greatly determined by age, such cases of "priorism" are not infrequent. They will be referred to again in the course of the discussion of the contents of the *Nei Ching*.

PHILOSOPHICAL FOUNDATIONS

The form in which the *Yellow Emperor's Canon of Internal Medicine* is written is quite remarkable for a textbook on the practice of medicine. It takes the form of dialogue between Huang Ti and his minister, Ch'i Po (歧 伯), in which the emperor generally poses the

33. See Appendix III for the translation of the preface written by Kao Pao-hêng and Lin I in 1078.

34. "The obscurity of Huang Ti's classic rendered necessary an elucidation of its difficulties, so in the third century B.C. the *Nan Ching* ("Difficult Classic") was written to solve eighty-one of its difficult questions. Eleven commentaries had been written on this previous to the Ming Dynasty, that is, before 1400 A.D. It might be said the difficulties have thereby been raised to the 11th degree." (Morse, *Chinese Medicine*, p. 41.)

35. In former times the commentary was interwoven with the text without the use of different types or sizes of ideographs. Later the commentary was distinguished by smaller types which are inserted in two vertical parallel columns into the original text.

questions and the minister branches into answers which are actually long discourses. This form of writing makes it possible to enlarge the scope of the work far beyond that of a medical textbook and to change it into a treatise on general ethics and regimen of life, and to include in it the prevailing Chinese religious beliefs. This combination is, as a matter of fact, the only way in which early Chinese medical thinking could be expressed, for medicine was but a part of philosophy and religion, both of which propounded oneness with nature, i.e. the universe.

Chinese religious philosophy, especially after the development of Taoism, Confucianism, and Buddhism, is rather complex, but for the purpose of facilitating the understanding of the *Nei Ching* it is sufficient to concentrate on three features which seem to have originated long before the development of any formal cult. These features, recurring with great frequency in the *Medical Canon*, are the concepts of (1) Tao, (2) Yin and Yang, and (3) the theory of the elements and, closely connected with it, the imposition upon the universe as well as upon man of a system of numbers among which the number five predominates.[36]

Tao

In an article on the foundations of Chinese medicine Dr. Edward H. Hume said: "To understand the older conceptions of medicine, it is essential to form a picture of the cosmogony, or philosophy of the origin of the world existing for centuries, but given form chiefly by Taoism."[37] But Lao-tzu (sixth century B.C.), the spiritual father of the movement of Taoism and supposedly the founder of natural philosophy, was only a manifestation of the much older

36. The Chinese do not possess any codified collection of early religious documents and nothing that can be compared to the holy scriptures of other peoples. Ancient Chinese literature is exclusively profane literature, but within it we find a number of texts which were collected and edited by Confucius and his disciples. Partly because of Confucius' editorship and partly because of their great age, these works receive the veneration that is usually bestowed upon texts which are held to be of divine origin. These ancient texts, collectively called the *Five Canons* (五 經), incidentally contain references to and descriptions of early Chinese religious thinking and practices. The philosophical and religious features, on which the theories of the *Nei Ching* are based, are frequently mentioned in the *Five Canons*, especially in the *I Ching* ("Book of Changes"), the *Shu Ching* ("Book of Government") and the *Shih Ching* ("Book of Songs"). See Wylie, *Notes on Chinese Literature*, pp. 1–6.

37. Edward H. Hume, "Some Foundations of Chinese Medicine," *Chinese Medical Journal*, LXI (Sept.–Oct., 1942), 296.

universalism. Lao-tzu neither created the word Tao nor gave it its specific meaning.[38] Dr. Heinrich Hackmann in his volume on Chinese philosophy even goes so far as to say: "The word Tao, which later became the shibboleth of a separate creed, Taoism, is basically a concept common to all Chinese and therefore retains its validity also in Confucianism and even in Buddhism. Tao is the key to the mysterious intermingling of 'Heaven and Earth,' Tao means the way and the method of maintaining the harmony between this world and the beyond, that is, by shaping earthly conduct to correspond completely with the demands of the other world."[39]

It is only logical that the Chinese, having for thousands of years before Lao-tzu and Confucius derived their livelihood from agriculture,[40] should have developed at an early time theoretical as well as practical foundations for their relationship with nature. The crystallization of this development was expressed by the concept of Tao, originally meaning the "Way." Since the entire universe followed one immutable course which became manifest through the change of night to day, through the recurrence of the seasons, through growth and decay, man in his utter dependence upon the universe could not do better than follow a way which was conceived after that of nature. The only manner in which man could attain the right Way, the Tao, was by emulating the course of the universe and complete adjustment to it. Thus man saw the universe endowed with a spirit that was indomitable in its strength and unforgiving towards disobedience.

Yet the ancient Chinese, although dependent upon the universe as a whole, realized that within nature itself there was a gradation of power: the earth was dependent upon heaven. When the fields were scorched and men waited for rain, when winter lingered and sun was needed to thaw the frozen earth, man saw that heaven was the more powerful and therefore made heaven his supreme deity. But Chinese imagination never personalized this higher being to the extent of speculating about its intrinsic qualities.[41] Heaven through its visible manifestations remained the ruler of the world

38. Otto Franke, "Die Chinesen" in Chantepie de la Saussure, *Religionsgeschichte* (Tübingen, 1925), Aufl. 4, Bd. I, pp. 195 ff.
39. Hackmann, *Chinesische Philosophie*, p. 26.
40. Herbert F. Rudd, *Chinese Social Origins* (Chicago, 1928), p. 3.
41. Wilhelm Grube, *Religion und Kultus der Chinesen* (Leipzig, 1910), pp. 27–31. See also W. Grube, "Religion der alten Chinesen" in *Religionsgeschichtliches Lesebuch*, ed. A. Bertholet (Tübingen, 1908), pp. 4 ff.

and united its Tao with that of the earth in order to complete the yearly cycle of nature; this was the example after which man formed his Tao.   Thus the concept of Tao, the Way, was subdivided into the Tao of Heaven, the Tao of the Earth, and the Tao of Man, one fitting into the other as an indivisible entity.[42]

The Theory of the Tao Applied to the Nei Ching

It was, of course, inevitable that Tao in its dual role as the supreme regulator of the universe and as the highest code of conduct should play an important part in early Chinese medical thought, which was so inextricably entwined with philosophical concepts.   This finds expression in the *Nei Ching*, where numerous references impress the reader that his health, and with it the highly desirable state of longevity, depended largely upon his own behaviour toward Tao. Longevity itself became to a certain degree a token of sainthood, since it was an indication that it had been achieved by the personal effort of complete adherence to Tao.   Thus in the initial chapter of the *Nei Ching* we read of a number of mythological sages who enjoyed eternal youth as a consequence of their adherence to Tao: "Those who follow Tao achieve the formula of perpetual youth and maintain a youthful body.   Although they are old in years they are still able to produce offspring."

This theme continues to discuss the particular efforts of each of the four groups of sages in their pursuit of the Tao.

Although the authors of the *Nei Ching* presuppose a definite knowledge on the part of the reader of the meaning of the word Tao and a certain familiarity with the methods of adherence to Tao, the second chapter does present an outline, according to which human conduct must vary according to the season.   Particular emphasis is achieved in this chapter by the enumeration of specific punishments which follow immediately upon each disobedience towards the laws of a season.   The references to Tao, numerous though they are throughout the *Nei Ching*, rarely discuss the Tao alone but generally in conjunction with the two component parts of the universe, the Yin and the Yang.

42. For a detailed description of the early concepts of Tao see J. J. M. de Groot, *Universismus, die Grundlage der Religion und Ethik, des Staatswesens und der Wissenschaften Chinas* (Berlin, 1918), pp. 1-23.

Yin and Yang

Although since earliest times heaven has been venerated as the supreme power, it was never credited with having created the world. Mythology has no place in the Chinese concept of creation; instead, the Chinese have groped towards a more scientific explanation of the cosmogony. According to Professor Alfred Forke, Lieh-tze, the oldest author who proposes a theory of creation, ". . . starts from chaos, in which the three primary elements of the universe—force, form and substance—were still undivided. This first stage is followed by a second, the great inception, when force becomes separated, then by a third, the great beginning, when form appears, and a fourth, the great homogeneity, when substance becomes visible. Then the light and pure substances rise above and form heaven, the heavier and coarser sink down and produce the earth."[43]

This concept of the division of substance into a lighter and a heavier part is one of the many forms which express the origin of the Chinese belief in a dual power. Even though the idea of the chaos—the first stage of the creation of the world—was later replaced by the Great Void, the Absolute, and then by the Great Unity or the Monad, the idea that each of these primary conditions divided into two and then reunited into one has survived.

The dual power that arose from the primary state was held to be the instigator of all change, for change was viewed as expression of duality, as an emergence of a second out of a first state. The two components of the dual power were designated as Yin and Yang. The two characters which stand for Yin and Yang have received a vast variety of interpretations, but by analyzing the ideographs themselves the original and basic meaning of the characters can be ascertained. A literal translation of the components that constitute the two characters result in the meaning of "the shady side of a hill" for Yin (陰) and "the sunny side of a hill" for Yang (陽).[44] Other interpretations see Yin and Yang as two banks of a river, one of which lies in the shade, the other exposed to the sun.[45] Dr. Otto Franke combines these two interpretations by stating that Yin represents the river bank that is shaded by a mountain, whereas

43. Forke, *World Conception of the Chinese*, p. 34.
44. Chalmers, *Structure of Chinese Characters*, p. 154, and Léon Wieger, *Leçons étymologiques* (Sienhsien, [1923?]), p. 265.
45. Hackmann, *Chinesische Philosophie*, p. 32.

Yang is that side of the river which is lighted by the sun.[46]   These three interpretations agree on the main issue, namely that Yin represents the shady, cloudy element, while Yang stands for the sunny and clear element.

Since Yin and Yang are supposed to be the primogenial elements from which the universe was evolved,[47] it was natural that they should be endowed with innumerable qualities.   But if we keep in mind their original meanings—cloudy and sunny—and their original functions—that of the creation of heaven and earth—we shall find that many of the additional connotations are either directly related to, or at least logically derived from the original concepts.

Yang stands for sun, heaven, day, fire, heat, dryness, light, and many other related subjects; Yang tends to expand, to flow upwards and outwards.   Yin stands for moon, earth, night, water, cold, dampness, and darkness; Yin tends to contract and to flow downwards.   As Heaven, Yang sends fertility in the form of sun (and rain) upon the earth; hence heaven's relation to earth is like that of man to wife—the man being Yang and the wife being Yin.   This classification of Yin and Yang was extended and applied to qualities which no longer bear a direct relationship to the original meaning of "shady" and "sunny," although the relationship can often be logically explained.   It would be impossible to enumerate even a small part of the alternatives Yin and Yang have come to represent. Nevertheless, a few examples showing their extension from the physical to the moral, from the concrete to the abstract, may be instructive.   Yang: motion, hence life; Yin: standstill, hence death.   Yang: high, hence noble; Yin: low, hence common.   Yang: good-beautiful; Yin: evil-ugly.   Further contrasts are: virtue-vice; order-confusion; reward-punishment; joy-sadness; wealth-poverty; health-disease.[48]

The fact that in these contrasts Yang represented the positive and Yin the negative side, must not be interpreted to mean that Yin was a "bad" and Yang a "good" principle.   It must always be borne in mind that Yin and Yang were conceived of as one entity and that both together were ever-present.   Day changed into night, light into darkness, spring and summer into fall and winter.   From these, the most striking and regular manifestations, it was deduced

46. Franke, "Die Chinesen," p. 197.
47. Forke, *World Conception of the Chinese*, p. 176.
48. *Ibid.*, pp. 188 ff.

that all happenings in nature as well as in human life were conditioned by the constantly changing relationship of these two cosmic regulators.   But the general application of this ever-present duality also led to the realization that neither of the components ever existed in an absolute state and the concept arose that within Yang there was contained Yin and within Yin there was contained Yang. The *Canon of Medicine* provides us with many examples of this interchange between Yin and Yang and of the duality preserved within a single thing.   The most concrete example of this duality is man. As a male, man belongs to Yang; as a female, man belongs to Yin. Yet both, male and female, are products of two primary elements, hence both qualities are contained in both sexes.

Yin and Yang in the Huang Ti Nei Ching Su Wên

In its concept of the creation of the universe the *Nei Ching* is in complete accord with the previously mentioned theories.   The following passages taken from chapters five and six are illustrative of the importance attributed to the two cosmic regulators:

"The principle of Yin and Yang is the basis of the entire universe.   It is the principle of everything in creation.   It brings about the transformation to parenthood; it is the root and source of life and death . . . .

"Heaven was created by an accumulation of Yang; the Earth was created by an accumulation of Yin.

"The ways of Yin and Yang are to the left and to the right.   Water and fire are the symbols of Yin and Yang.   Yin and Yang are the source of power and the beginning of everything in creation.

"Yang ascends to Heaven; Yin descends to Earth.   Hence the universe (Heaven and Earth) represents motion and rest, controlled by the wisdom of nature.   Nature grants the power to beget and to grow, to harvest and to store, to finish and to begin anew."

The constant interaction of the two basic elements is described in the following paragraph:

"Everything in creation is covered by Heaven and supported by the Earth. When nothing has as yet come forth the Earth is called: 'the place where Yin dwells'; it is also known as the Yin within the Yin.   Yang supplies that which is upright, while Yin acts as a ruler of Yang."

In later chapters are offered detailed descriptions as to the interrelation of Yin and Yang within the human body.   Since this interrelationship, based upon a complex system and a fixed terminology, is constantly referred to throughout the entire work, it might be well to explain it in detail in order to facilitate the understanding of the passages that allude to it.

Man, according to the system propounded in the *Nei Ching*, was subdivided into a lower region, a middle region, and an upper region, and each of these regions was again subdivided three times, each subdivision containing an element of heaven, an element of earth, and an element of man.   This scheme of subdivisions was concurrent with another scheme according to which each of the three main subdivisions was held to be composed of one part of Yin and one part of Yang; i.e., the human body was regarded as consisting of three parts of Yin and three parts of Yang.   Since treatment of a specific disease or a specific organ depended largely on its location within a particular part of Yin or Yang, knowledge of these subdivisions was very important for diagnosis as well as for treatment.   The names for the various regions which occur with great frequency through the entire work are as follows:[49]

Yang		*Yin*	
(太 陽)	The Great Yang	(太 陰)	The Great Yin
(少 陽)	The Lesser Yang	(少 陰)	The Lesser Yin
(陽 明)	The 'Sunlight'	(厥 陰)	The Absolute Yin

In chapter twenty-two we find a description of the relationship of each subdivision to its particular organ, as well as of the relationship of the organs to each other and the relationship between the various subdivisions.   From this description the following diagram can be evolved:

The Absolute Yin (厥 陰) includes the liver
The Lesser Yang (少 陽) includes the gall
                           bladder
           } These two organs are closely connected

The Lesser Yin (少 陰) includes the heart
The Great Yang (太 陽) includes the small
                           intestines
           } These two organs are closely connected

The Great Yin (太 陰) includes the spleen
The 'Sunlight' (陽 明) includes the stomach
           } These two organs are closely connected

---

49. See chapter 20.   It is very difficult to translate these conceptions adequately.   All, except the "Absolute Yin," are literal translations of the characters; the Absolute Yin is as close to a literal translation as the character 厥 permits.   The six names should not be considered for their meaning but only as specifications for each of the six regions.

The Great Yin	(太 陰) includes the lungs	These two organs are closely connected
The 'Sunlight'	(陽 明) includes the lower intestines	

The Lesser Yin	(少 陰) includes the kidneys	These two organs are closely connected
The 'Sunlight'	(陽 明) includes the bladder	

The cosmic relationship of Yang and Yin as light and darkness is, in the *Nei Ching*, carried over into the physical structure of man. In chapter 5 we find the sentence: "Yin is active within and acts as a guardian of Yang; Yang is active on the outside and acts as a regulator of Yin." Thus, in regard to the human body, Yang and Yin corresponded to the surface and the interior respectively.[50] Moreover, since both elements also existed within the body, this relationship in regard to the organs was compared to that of a coat and its lining.[51]

As can be expected, the affinity of Yin and Yang to each other was held to have a decisive influence upon man's health. Perfect harmony between the two primogenial elements meant health; disharmony or undue preponderance of one element brought disease and death. This is explained in chapter 5, where the process of aging is attributed to the waning of the Yin element within the body. But man is not helplessly exposed to the whims of Yin and Yang. Man had received the doctrine of Tao as a means of maintaining perfect balance and to secure for himself health and long life. In the *I Ching*, the most ancient of the Five Canons,[52] it is said: 一陽一陰之謂道; translated by de Groot this sentence reads: "The Yang and the Yin of the Universe are called Tao."[53] This knowledge of Tao and of the workings of Yin and Yang was considered even strong enough to counteract the effect of age. Thus we find it said in the *Nei Ching* that "those who have the true wisdom remain strong, while those who have no wisdom grow old and feeble." The ideal age for man expounded by the *Nei Ching* was one hundred years.[54] In order to impress their readers with the desirability of long life and the necessity of following the Tao, the authors of the *Nei Ching* made use of the impressive device of 'priorism' and described

50. See chapter 4 of translation.
51. See chapter 24 of translation.
52. See footnote 31.
53. de Groot, *Universismus*, p. 8.
54. See chapter 1 of translation.

sages of ancient and medieval[55] times who followed Tao and thus achieved longevity. All these sages, of whom there was an entire hierarchy based upon the remoteness of the time in which they lived, fulfilled their Tao in a similar manner: they lived in harmony with heaven and earth, Yin and Yang, and the four seasons.

It is not at all surprising to find the four seasons mentioned in connection with Yin and Yang; the seasons were looked upon merely as the result of the interaction of the two forces which stood for sun and moon, heat and cold, dryness and humidity. The Tao which was required of the Chinese in regard to the four seasons is the same mode of life required of any agricultural people at any time and anywhere in the world; and it is stated very simply in chapter 6 of the *Nei Ching*:

"Planting and begetting are in accord with spring; growing and cultivating are in accord with summer; gathering in the harvest is in accord with fall; and the storing of the crop is in accord with winter."

The Five Elements and the System of Numbers

In the previous sections, we traced the close connection between Tao, Yin and Yang, and the four seasons, and we learned the meaning of Tao in regard to the four seasons. However, for the analysis of Tao in regard to Yin and Yang it is necessary to break down the concept of Yin and Yang into more tangible components. These tangible components, or creations, of Yin and Yang are the five elements.

55. This mention of sages of ancient and medieval times has by some authors been accepted as conclusive proof that the *Nei Ching* was composed as late as the third century B.C. Sang Yueh(桑 悅), an editor of the *Su Wên* (素 問), ". . . holds the opinion that the book was not from the pen of Huang Ti, for the terms 'ancient' and 'medieval' were employed which is conclusive proof that it must have been written about the time of early Ch'in or the Warring States." (See Wong and Wu, *History of Chinese Medicine*, p. 17). Yet, if it was possible to use the terms "ancient" and "medieval" in the third century B.C., it can be surmised that they were also used in earlier times when reference was made to previous periods. The Chinese tendency to the use of priorism is ancient and closely connected with ancestor worship. When Confucius created a picture of antiquity and of ancient rulers, which corresponded—and was supposed to correspond—less to historical truth than to an ideal established for the princes and their people, his use of "priorism" would not have met with such success had the device not been an accepted one. According to Dr. Franke ("Die Chinesen," p. 207), it is dangerous to move the ideals of a people into a great past, for it interferes with man's normal urge to expect and to work for improvement in the future. The tendency towards priorism becomes even more harmful if historical truth about recent events is obliterated and a golden age alone is worshipped.

According to Dr. Alfred Forke, "the theory of the five elements (五 行) is no doubt of Chinese origin and its existence in ancient times proved by many old documents."[56] The essence of this ancient tradition is that Yin and Yang, in addition to exerting their dual power, subdivided into water, fire, metal, wood, and earth. Man, who was said to be the product of heaven and earth by the inter-action of Yin and Yang, also contains, therefore, the five elements. This close relationship between the five elements and the human body was also extended to human actions.

The sequence of the five elements varies according to the view-point with which they are enumerated, for they are said to vanquish one another and to produce one another. The *Nei Ching* explains the mutual victories of the elements in the following manner: "*Wood* brought in contact with metal is felled; *fire* brought in contact with water is extinguished; *earth* brought in contact with wood is pene-trated; *metal* brought in contact with fire is dissolved; *water* brought in contact with earth is halted."[57] Thus the sequence of subjuga-tion is:

> metal subjugates wood
> water   "   fire
> wood   "   earth
> fire   "   metal
> earth   "   water

The sequence of creation is:

> metal creates water
> water   "   wood
> wood   "   fire
> fire   "   earth
> earth   "   metal

The five elements were also distributed over the seasons, i.e., each element was attached to a particular season; wood belonged to spring, fire belonged to summer, metal belonged to fall and water belonged to winter. While the element that belonged to one season was at its height, the element connected with the previous season was waning, the element connected with the following season was

56. Forke, *World-Conception of the Chinese*, p. 237.
57. See translation, chapter 25.

waxing, and the fourth element was in a temporary eclipse. According to this scheme each element was alive for nine months—strongest during its particular season—and inactive for the three months of its eclipse.

Each season was thought to originate from one point of the compass; hence the element of each season was also the element of the direction from which the season originated. Yet, since there were five elements but only four seasons and four directions, one additional season, the last month of summer or "Late Summer" (季 夏) and one additional direction, the Center, were created to serve where complete numerical concordance was imperative.

These numerical concordances, which Dr. Heinrich Hackmann calls the most poignant symbol of mythical thinking,[58] are evident through most of ancient Chinese literature. The *Nei Ching*, however, in its attempt to schematize the functioning of the body, established its theories almost entirely upon systems of numbers which by their sheer weight of parallelism seemed to explain the workings of the universe and the human body. In the first chapter of the *Nei Ching* we find a striking description of the development of the female and the male body based upon the numbers seven and eight.

The development of the woman: at the age of seven her teeth and hair grow longer; at fourteen she begins to menstruate and can bear children; at twenty-one she is fully grown and her physical condition is at its best; at twenty-eight her muscles are firm, her body is flourishing; at thirty-five her face begins to wrinkle and her hair begins to fall; at forty-two her arteries begin to harden, and her hair turns white; at forty-nine she ceases to menstruate and she is no longer able to bear children.

The development of the man: at the age of eight his hair grows long and he changes his teeth; at sixteen he begins to secrete semen; at twenty-four his testicles are fully developed and he has reached his full height; at thirty-two his muscles are firm; at forty his testicles begin to weaken, he begins to lose his hair, and his teeth begin to decay; at forty-eight his masculine vigor is exhausted, his face becomes wrinkled and his hair turns gray; at fifty-six his secretions diminish and his testicles deteriorate.

In this rigid scheme no allowance of any kind is made for possible

58. Hackmann, *Chinesische Philosophie*, p. 35.

individual differences from these two scales of development. The numbers and their multiples constitute the law for the growth and decline of man. A similar but much more complicated law is enforced by the number five, which serves to integrate man's body and emotions into the universe. The number five was chosen because the basis of this system is furnished by the five elements. As was mentioned above, a concordance had been established between each of the elements and one particular season and direction. This concordance was extended to flavors, odors, climates, musical notes, grains, animals, many other groups, each of which contained five components, and—significantly—to the physical organs.

The *Nei Ching*, as mentioned before, abounds in references to such concordances, the knowledge of which was taken for granted by the author. The following diagrams, assembled from many references to the number five system, may serve to explain the text itself:

	Yang	*Yang*		*Yin*	*Yin*
SEASON	Spring	Summer	Late Summer (季夏) Long Summer (長夏)	Fall	Winter
DIRECTION	East	South	Center	West	North
CLIMATE	Wind	Heat	Humidity	Dryness	Cold
VISCERA	Liver	Heart	Spleen	Lungs	Kidneys
ELEMENT	Wood	Fire	Earth	Metal	Water
COLOR	Green	Red	Yellow	White	Black
MUSICAL NOTE	*chio* (角)	*chih* (徵)	*kung* (宮)	*shang* (商)	*yü* (羽)
NUMBER	8	7	5	9	6
FLAVOR	Sour	Bitter	Sweet	Pungent	Salt
ODOR	Rancid	Scorched	Fragrant	Rotten	Putrid
SOUND	Shout	Laugh	Sing	Weep	Groan
EMOTIONS	Anger	Joy	Sympathy	Grief	Fear
ORIFICES	Eyes	Ears	Nose	Mouth	"Lower orifices"
ANIMALS	Fowl	Sheep	Ox	Horse	Pig
GRAINS	Wheat	Glutinous millet	Millet	Rice	Beans (peas)
PLANET	Jupiter	Mars	Saturn	Venus	Mercury
BOWELS	Gall bladder	Small intestine	Stomach	Large intestine	3 burning spaces and bladder
TISSUES	Ligaments	Arteries	Muscles	Skin and hair	Bones

Three of the groups mentioned in this chart of concordances require some explanation:

The musical notes are the five notes that constituted the ancient pentatonic scale.

Dr. Alfred Forke explains the reason for the selection of the numbers as follows: "The ordinary numerals attached to the elements in the *Liki* ["Book of Rites" and one of the Five Canons], are said to refer to the ten stages or turns in which originally the Five Elements were evolved from *Yin* and *Yang*, of Heaven and Earth.   Tai T'ing-huai states that:

1st. Heaven engendered water.	2ndly. Earth engendered fire.
3rdly. Heaven engendered wood.	4thly. Earth engendered metal.
5thly. Heaven engendered earth.	6thly. Earth completed water.
7thly. Heaven completed fire.	8thly. Earth completed wood.
9thly. Heaven completed metal.	10thly. Earth completed earth.

Now all elements are given the numbers of their completion—water-6, fire-7, wood-8, metal-9—except earth, which bears the number of its generation, because . . . generation is the principal thing for earth.   This reason is as singular as the whole theory of this creation in ten stages."[59]

In the general grouping of the orifices, the eyes and the ears belong to the region of Yang, and the mouth and the "lower orifices" (anus and urethra) belong to the region of Yin.   But taken by themselves, the eyes, the ears, the nose and the mouth are organs of Yang and only the lower orifices are organs of Yin.[60]

The table of main concordances serves as a basis for a number of fixed relationships:[61]

The five fluid secretions as connected with the viscera:

> perspiration is connected with the heart
> mucus   is connected with the lungs
> tears   are connected with the liver
> saliva   is connected with the spleen
> spittle   is connected with the kidneys

59. Forke, *World Concepion of the Chinese*, pp. 284–285.
60. See translation, chapter 3.
61. See translation, chapter 23.

The five climates as they affect the viscera:[62]

> heat   injures the heart
> cold   injures the lungs
> wind   injures the liver
> humidity injures the spleen
> dryness injures the kidneys

The controls exerted by the viscera:[63]

> the heart   controls the pulse
> the lungs   control the skin
> the liver   controls the muscles
> the spleen controls the flesh
> the kidneys control the bones

The effect of the flavors upon the body:[64]

> excess of salty flavor   hardens the pulse
> excess of bitter flavor withers the skin
> excess of pungent flavor knots the muscles
> excess of sour flavor   toughens the flesh
> excess of sweet flavor   causes aches in the bones

The five spiritual resources as controlled by the viscera:

> the liver   controls the soul (魂)
> the heart   controls the spirit (神)
> the spleen controls the ideas (意)
> the lungs   control the inferior spirit or animal spirit (魄)
> the kidneys control the will (志)

The effects of the five flavors:[65]

> the pungent flavor has a dispersing effect
> the sour flavor   has a gathering (stringent) effect
> the sweet flavor   has a retarding effect
> the bitter flavor has a strengthening effect
> the salty flavor   has a softening effect

The injuries caused by the climate of one season become manifest in the following season:[66]

---

62. See translation, chapter 23.
63. See translation, chapter 23.
64. See translation, chapter 10.
65. See translation, chapter 20.
66. See translation, chapter 5.

The injuries caused by the cold of winter cause a recurrence of the illness in spring

The injuries caused by the wind of spring make people
unable to retain food in summer

The injuries caused by the heat of summer cause intermittent fever in fall

The injuries caused by the humidity of fall cause a cough
in winter

Other interrelationships are:[67]

The heart is connected with the pulse and rules over the
kidneys

The lungs are connected with the skin and rule over the
heart

The liver is connected with the muscles and rules over
the lungs

The spleen is connected with the flesh and rules over the
lungs

The kidneys are connected with the bones and rule over
the spleen

The liver nourishes the muscles; the muscles strengthen
the heart

The heart nourishes the blood; the blood strengthens the
spleen

The spleen nourishes the flesh; the flesh strengthens the
lungs

The lungs nourish the skin and the hair; the skin and the
hair strengthen the kidneys

The kidneys nourish the bones and the marrow; the bones
and the marrow strengthen the liver[68]

The Celestial Stems

The relationship between the points of the compass and the
seasons was based not only upon the elements they had in common,
but also upon an ancient device that measured time and denoted the
heavenly directions. This device is called the "Celestial Stems"
(天 干). There are ten celestial stems whose eternal cycle represents

67. See translation, chapter 10.
68. See translation, chapter 5.

the passage of time.   In the *Nei Ching* they appear in dual combinations and serve as alternative designations of the seasons, although, strictly speaking, they are only the two signs for the first two days of a season of seventy-two days.   Thus we find the following combinations:[69]

Season	Celestial Stem	Element
fall	(庚 辛)	metal
winter	(壬 癸)	wood
spring	(甲 乙)	water
summer	(丙 丁)	fire
long summer⎱ late summer⎰	(戊 巳)	earth

ANATOMICAL AND PHYSIOLOGICAL CONCEPTS OF THE NEI CHING

In the preceding sections dealing with Yin and Yang and the five elements, and in the charts illustrating the various concordances, it was shown how closely the Chinese concepts of the structure of the human body are connected with the Chinese theories of cosmogony.   As a result of this great stress upon schematization we receive a picture of human anatomy that is highly stylized and of little practical significance.   Even if it were true that, as Dr. E. T. Hsieh states, "in the beginning the science of anatomy in China was based upon actual dissection of the body,"[70] the findings were not exploited scientifically, but, as Dr. Lockhart, an English missionary and surgeon, so pertinently summed up, ". . . just as if some person had seen some imperfect dissection of the interior of the body, and then sketched from memory a representation of the organs, filling up parts that were obscure out of his own imaginings, and portraying what, according to his own opinion ought to be, rather than what they in reality are."[71]

According to the *Nei Ching* man has five "viscera" (臟) and six "bowels" (腑).   The viscera are the heart, the spleen, the lungs, the liver, and the kidneys.   They are credited with the capacity of storing, but not of elimination.   They determine the functions of all the other parts of the body, including the bowels, and also of the

69. For additional information on the celestial stems see de Groot, *Universismus*, pp. 320–321, 233.   The ideographs for the celestial stems cannot be translated; they are usually written in Chinese characters, since too frequent use of romanization causes lack of clarity.
70. E. T. Hsieh, "A Review of Ancient Chinese Anatomy," *Anatomical Record*, XX (1921), 123.
71. William R. Morse, *Chinese Medicine* (New York, 1934), pp. 69–70.

腎居十四椎各開一寸半重一觔二兩主存志

其臟獨二枚左屬相火右屬眞水於卦爲坎坎

中滿其間爲

命門眞火○

難經曰左爲

腎右爲命門

命門者男子

以存精女子以繫胞

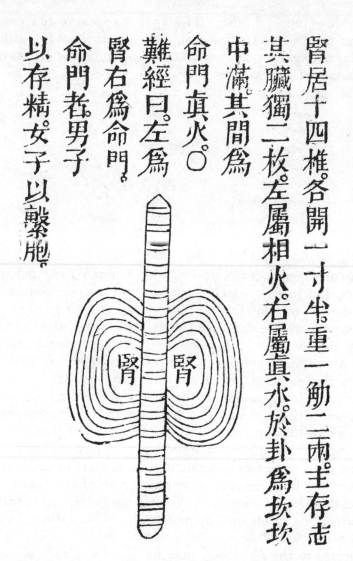

FIG. 1. THE KIDNEYS

From *Ling Shu Su Wên Chieh Yao Ch'ien Chu*, compiled by Ch'ên Hsiu-yüan (also known as Ch'ên Nien-shih) of the Ch'ing dynasty

府焦三陽少手

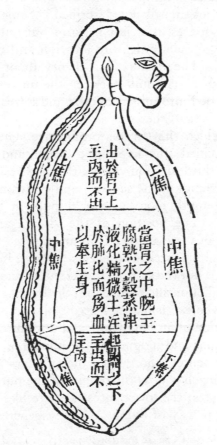

FIG. 2. THE THREE BURNING SPACES

From: *Ling Shu Su Wên Chieh Yao*

spiritual resources and emotions. The six bowels, which are held
to have the capacity of elimination but not of storing, are the gall
bladder, the stomach, the lower intestines, the small intestines, and
the three foci, or three burning spaces (三 焦). The question as to
location and function of this latter organ (or organs) has given rise
to various interpretations. In the *Nei Ching* the function of the
three burning spaces is compared to that of a sewage system of the
body, while their location is not described. Some sources maintain
that the burning spaces exist not in form but only in name, while
others attributed to them a definite location and the consistency of
fatty membranes. The most explicit theory about the three burning
spaces considers them as a link between the universe and man, and
sees them subdivided into upper, middle and lower parts controlling
corresponding regions of the body.[72]

The order in which the various organs are generated—or rather
animated—is specified: the liver in the first and second months;
the spleen in the third and fourth months; the head in the fifth and
sixth months; the lungs in the seventh and eighth months; the heart
in the ninth and tenth months; the kidneys in the eleventh and
twelfth months.[73] The position of the viscera and the bowels is
compared to that of various officials in an empire: "The heart is like
the minister of the monarch who excels through insight and understanding; the lungs are the symbol of the interpretation and conduct
of the official jurisdiction and regulation; the liver has the functions of
a military leader who excels in his strategic planning; the gall bladder
occupies the position of an important and upright official who excels
through his decisions and judgment; the middle of the thorax is like
the official of the center who guides the subjects in their joys and
pleasures; the stomach acts as the official of the public granaries and
grants the five tastes; the lower intestines are like the officials who
propagate the right way of living and they generate evolution and

72. Hsieh, "Review of Ancient Chinese Anatomy," pp. 111–113, and Morse, *Chinese Medicine*, pp. 68–69.

73. Translation, chapter 16. It is difficult to establish the basis for the order of the animation
of the viscera, for this order does not agree with the generally applied concordance,
according to which the sequence would be: liver, heart, spleen, lungs, kidneys. It is
possible that the reason for the transversion of the spleen, the lungs and the heart, was
due to the mistake of a copyist. It is evident, however, that the head was added to the
five viscera in order to enable the author to divide the year into groups of two-month
periods.

肝居膈下上着脊之九椎下是經多血少氣其

合筋也其榮爪也主存魂開竅於目其系上絡

心肺下亦無竅〇難經

曰肝重四觔四兩左三

葉右四葉凡七葉〇滑

氏曰肝之爲臟其治在

左其臟在右脅石腎之

前並胃着炎目之第九椎

肝

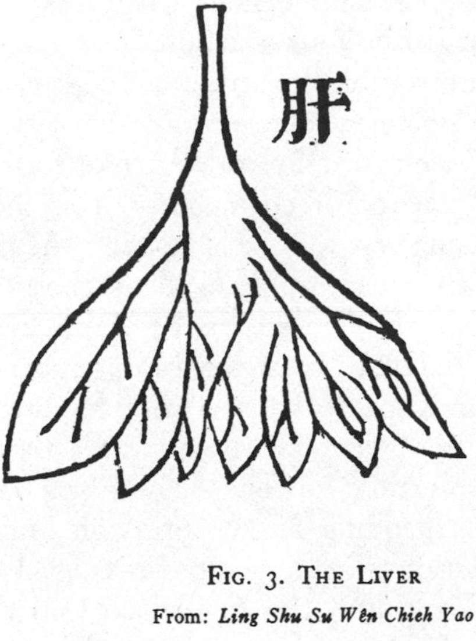

FIG. 3. THE LIVER

From: *Ling Shu Su Wên Chieh Yao*

change; the small intestines are like the officials who are entrusted with riches and they create changes of the physical substance; the kidneys are like the officials who do energetic work and they excel through their ability; the three burning spaces are like the officials who plan the construction of ditches and sluices and they create waterways; the groins and the bladder are like the magistrates of a region, they store the overflow and the fluid secretions which serve to regulate vaporization. These twelve officials should not fail to assist one another."[74]

In addition to the viscera and bowels represented as the ministers, the *Nei Ching* recognizes as storing organs the brain, the marrow, the bones, all of which were held to have been produced by the earth and hence belong to *Yin*.

The measurements of time and the number of the components of the body are held to agree perfectly. The three hundred and sixty-five days of the year are matched by the theory that man consists of three hundred and sixty-five parts. The twelve months are paralleled by the twelve main vessels (or ducts), and the four main arteries correspond to the four seasons.

It is difficult, if not impossible, to draw a dividing line between the anatomical and physiological concepts of the *Nei Ching*. The organs are described for their function rather than for their location and structure, and the theory of cosmogony, i.e., the continuous interaction of Yin and Yang, the four seasons, and the five elements, dominates the theories on structure as well as those on function. Some of the organs are ruled by Yin, others by Yang, and the viscera and bowels are either in a state of harmony or of opposition, depending upon the lack or abundance of the two primary forces. Yin was credited with the production of perspiration while Yang was thought to cause dry heat. Perspiration, however, could originate from any one of the five viscera, depending on the exertion forced upon the particular organ. Digestion was held to be caused by the collaboration of Yin and Yang and the five viscera in the following manner: the food enters the stomach; its essence flows into the liver and from there its vital forces go into the muscles, its putrid gases ascend to the heart and its essence reaches the pulse, and finally its bulk descends by way of the anus. Drink enters the stomach

74. Translation, chapter 8.

難經曰。膽在肝之
短葉間重三兩三
銖長三寸盛精汁
三合。○是經多血
少氣。○華元化曰
膽者中清之府號
曰將軍○主守而
不瀉

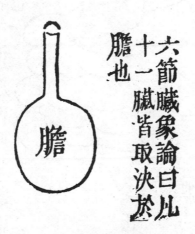

膽也

六節臟象論曰凡
十一臟皆取決於

FIG. 4. THE GALL BLADDER
From: *Ling Shu Su Wên Chieh Yao*

經曰大腸重二觔十二兩肛門重十二兩○按

腸者以其迴疊也廣腸者卽迴腸之更大也直

腸者又廣腸之末節也下連肛門是爲穀道後

陰一名魄門皆大腸也

上口

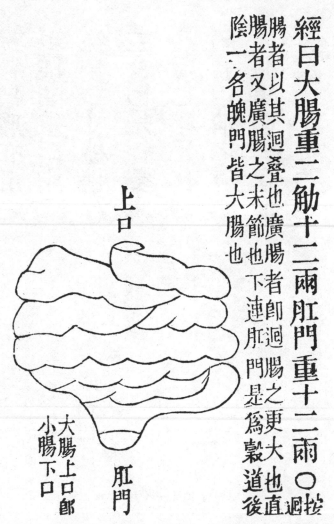

大腸上口卽
小腸下口

肛門

FIG. 5. THE LARGE INTESTINES

From: *Ling Shu Su Wên Chieh Yao*

清濁水液滲

人膀胱滓穢

流入大腸。○

是經多血少

氣。○難經曰

小腸重二觔

十四兩。

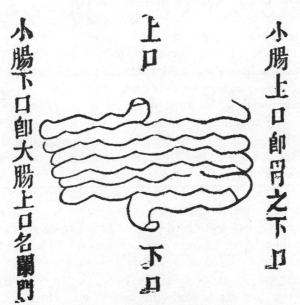

小腸下口卽大腸上口名闌門

上口

下口

小腸上口卽胃之下口

FIG. 6. THE SMALL INTESTINES

From: *Ling Shu Su Wên Chieh Yao*

then turns into secretion, the essence of which enters the spleen. The spleen in turn sends its secretions to the lungs, from which they descend into the bladder. Yin and Yang were also held to move about in the twelve main ducts and to determine the contents of the subsidiary vessels, which were thought to be filled with air and blood. Circulation of air and blood is frequently mentioned, yet its system is not described in detail, but held to be subordinate to the workings of Yin and Yang.

One of the most detailed accounts of the functions of the blood and its effect upon the various parts of the body reads as follows: "The four limbs and their eight flexible joints [elbows, knees, wrists and ankles] are in use from early morning until late at night. When people lie down to rest the blood flows back to the liver. When the liver receives the blood it strengthens the vision.[75] When the feet receive blood it strengthens the footsteps. When the palms of the hands receive blood the hands can be used to grasp. When the fingers receive blood they can be used to carry. When a person is exposed to the wind, either lying down to rest or walking about, his blood will be affected; the blood then coagulates within the flesh and the result is numbness within the hands and the feet. When the blood coagulates within the pulse it ceases to circulate beneficially. When the blood coagulates within the feet it causes pains and chills."[76] A direct relationship between the blood and the heart is recognized, but only as a part of a formula based on the number five, according to which the pulse is connected with the eyes, the marrow is connected with the brain, the muscles are connected with the joints, and the breath is connected with the lungs.

The following selections from the *Nei Ching* are illustrative of the theories on which these connections are based: "The East creates the wind; the wind creates the wood; the wood creates the sour flavor; the sour flavor strengthens the liver; the liver nourishes the muscles; the muscles strengthen the heart; and the liver governs the eyes. The eyes see the mystery of Heaven and discover Tao among mankind.

"Upon earth there are transformation and change, which produce the five flavors. The attainment of Tao produces wisdom while the

75. According to the basic system of correlations, the eyes are connected with the liver.
76. See translation, chapter 10.

下。其與橫膜相粘而黃脂裹者心也脂漫之外

有細筋膜如絲與心相連者心包也此謬爲是

凡言無形者非。○又按靈蘭秘典論有十二官

獨少心包一官而多膻

中者臣使之官喜樂出

焉一節今考心包腑居

膈上經始胸中。正値膻中之所位居相火代君

行令實臣使也此一官者其卽此經之謂歟。

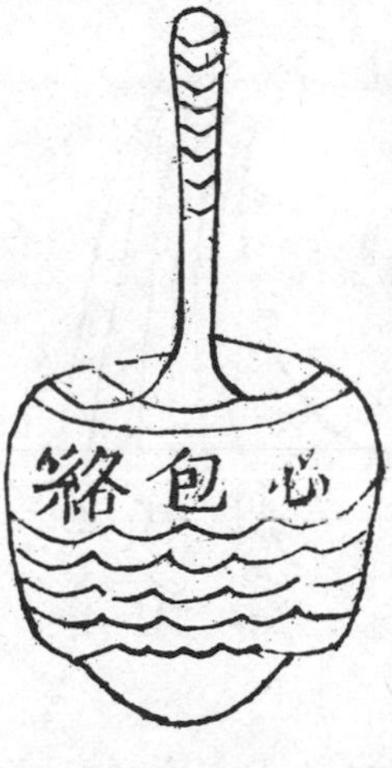

FIG. 7. THE PERICARDIUM

From: *Ling Shu Su Wên Chieh Yao*

有竅多寡不同心導引天真之氣下無透竅土
通乎舌只有四系以通四臟頭外有赤黃裹脂
是為心包絡心
不有膈膜與脊
脊周迴相著遮
蔽濁氣使不得
上薰心肺所謂
膻中也。

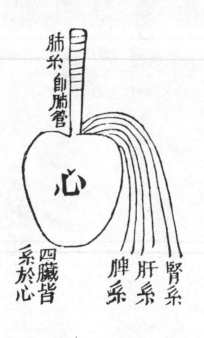

肺糸即肺管

心

四臟皆
系於心

腎系
肝系
脾系

FIG. 8. THE HEART

The thin lines pointing below indicate the connection of the heart with (from right to left) the kidneys, the liver, and the spleen. The tube leading into the heart from above forms the connection with the lungs and the trachea.

From: *Ling Shu Su Wên Chieh Yao*

有言其有上口無下
口有言上下俱有口
者皆非。○是經多血
少氣。○難經曰膀胱
重九兩二銖縱廣九
寸盛溺九升九合口
廣二寸半。

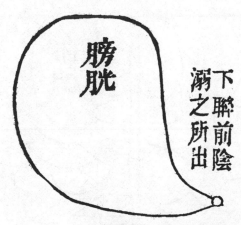

膀胱

下聯前陰
溺之所出

FIG. 9. THE BLADDER
From: *Ling Shu Su Wên Chieh Yao*

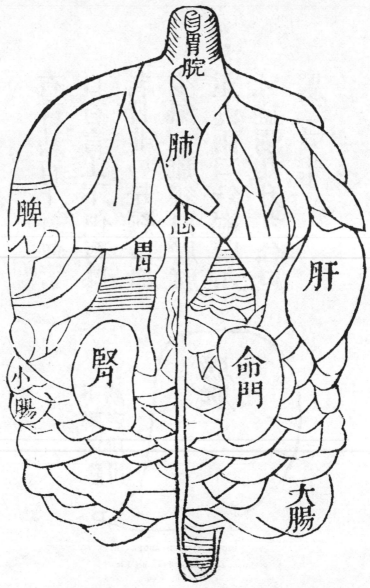

Fig. 10. Position of the Five Viscera, the Stomach, the Large Intestines, and the Small Intestines

The kidney is indicated as the seat of the imaginary organ, the 'Gate of Life'

From: *Ling Shu Su Wên Chieh Yao*

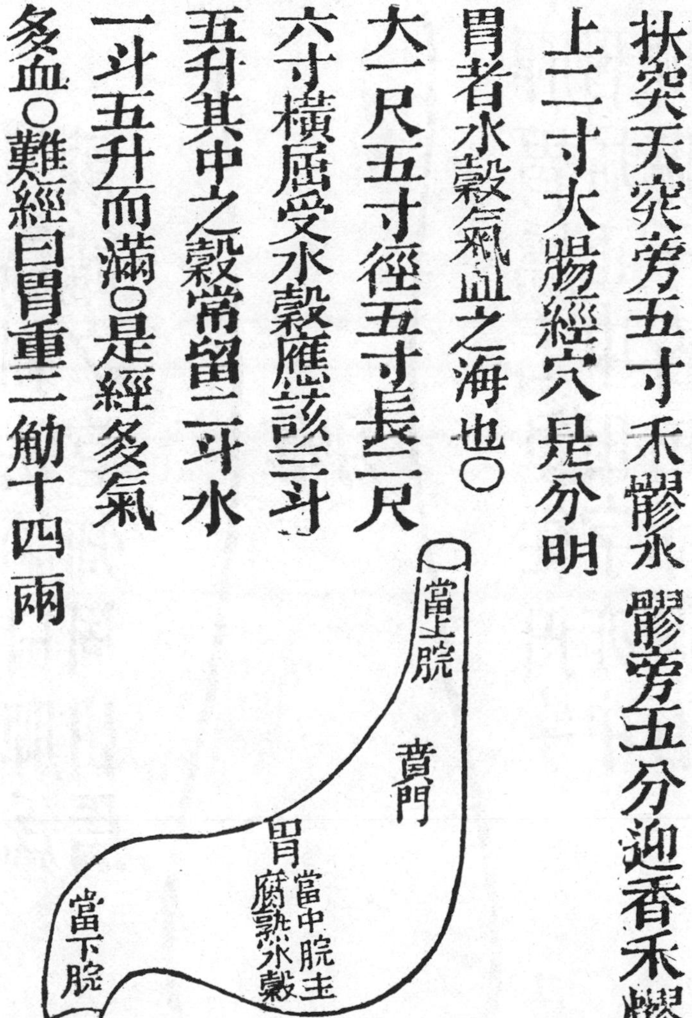

多血○難經曰胃重二觔十四兩
一斗五升而滿○是經多氣
五升其中之穀常留二斗水
六寸橫屈受水穀雁該三斗
大一尺五寸徑五寸長二尺
胃者水穀氣血之海也○
上二寸大腸經穴 是分明
扶突天突旁五寸禾髎水 髎旁五分迎香禾髎

當上脘
賁門
胃
當中脘主
腐熟水穀
當下脘

FIG. 11. THE STOMACH

From: *Ling Shu Su Wên Chieh Yao*

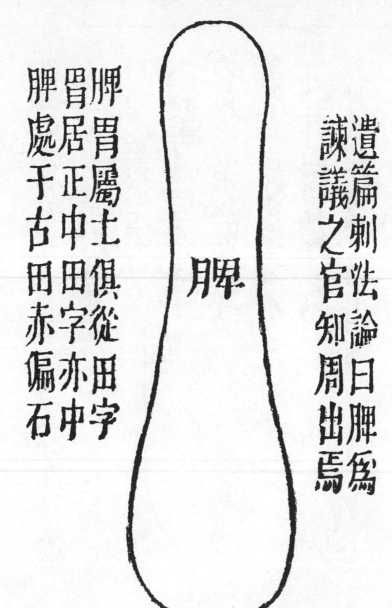

脾處于古田赤偏石

胃居正中田字亦中

脾胃屬土俱從田字

脾

遺篇刺法論曰脾爲

諫議之官知周出焉

FIG. 12. THE SPLEEN

From: *Ling Shu Su Wên Chieh Yao*

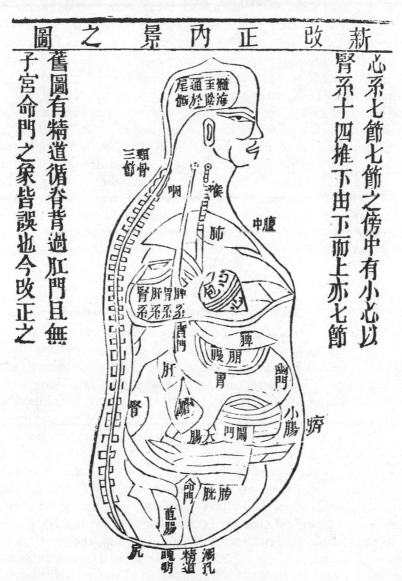

新改正內景之圖

心系七節七節之傍中有小心以
腎系十四椎下出下而上亦七節

舊圖有精道循脊背過肛門且無
子宮命門之象皆誤也今改正之

FIG. 13. THE INTERNAL ORGANS

From: *I Tsung Pi Tu,* compiled about 1575 A.D.

supernatural powers spring from the mysterious. The supernatural powers create wind in Heaven and they create wood upon earth. Within the body they create muscles and of the five viscera they create the liver. Of the colors they create the green color and of the musical notes they create the note *chio* (角). They give to the human voice the ability to form a shouting sound. In times of excitement and change they grant the capacity for control. Of the orifices they create the eyes; of the flavors they create the sour flavor, and of the emotions they create anger.

"Anger is injurious to the liver, but sympathy counteracts anger. Wind is injurious to the muscles, but heat and drought counteract the wind. The sour flavor is injurious to the muscles, but the pungent flavor counteracts the sour flavor."[77]

Similar correlations are also established for South, West and North.

DIAGNOSIS

The chief means of diagnosis employed in the *Nei Ching* is the examination of the pulse. All other methods of determining disease are only subsidiary to palpation and used mainly in connection with it. The theory of the pulse is based upon the various stages of interaction between Yin and Yang and upon the crasis or dyscrasia of the five elements. The correct balance between Yin and Yang and the harmonious mixture of the elements cause health; lack of balance and disharmony cause disease. The system of palpation propounded by the *Nei Ching*[78] was believed to be effective in the diagnosis of the nature and location of any kind of disease. The basis of this practice was the belief that the pulse actually consisted of six pulses, i.e., three sets of pulses on each hand, each connected with a particular part of the body and each able to record even the minutest pathological changes taking place within the body.

In the complicated process of taking the pulse, the physician had to consider many factors. In order to find an auspicious moment for his undertaking he had to decide which of the ten celestial stems

77. See translation, chapter 5.
78. The *Nei Ching* is only one of a great number of books dealing with the doctrine of the pulse. The most famous of these books is the *Meh Ching* or "Classic of the Pulse," written by Wang Shu-ho, around 280 A.D.

had started the first month of the year, because their constellation determined the day on which the examination was to take place. The best time of the day for the taking of the pulse was considered to be the very early morning, when the physician himself was still cool and collected, and "when the breath of Yin has not yet begun to stir and when the breath of Yang has not yet begun to diffuse, when food and drink have not yet been taken, when the twelve main vessels are not yet abundant, . . . when vigor and energy are not yet exerted."[79]

The procedure of palpation differed according to the sex of the patient: if it was a woman her right pulses had to be taken first; if it was a man his left pulses had to be examined first.[80] The seasons too were held to influence the pulse beats to a considerable extent: "In spring the pulse is dominated by the liver, in summer the pulse is dominated by the heart, in fall the pulse is dominated by the lungs, and in winter the pulse is dominated by the kidneys." The pulse of the spleen, however, is not related to any season, but to the earth, for "the spleen is a solitary organ, but it irrigates the four others. . . ."[81]

Thus the physician must know the normal sounds of the pulse beats of each of the five viscera and their respective changes during the five seasons, and he must be able to interpret the slightest aberration from the normal sound for the pathological change it represents. Furthermore, each of the three pulses on each hand was subdivided into an internal and an external pulse, and by means of this subdivision all parts of the body in addition to the viscera could be examined. Moreover, the three different qualities of Yin and Yang (the great Yang, the lesser Yang, the 'sunlight' and the great Yin, the lesser Yin, and the absolute Yin) were thought to be palpable at each of the twelve subdivisions of the pulse.

The task of the physician was further complicated by the fact

79. See translation, chapter 17.
80. See translation, chapter 15. In chapter 15 Wang Ping, the commentator, furnishes a basis for the explanation of this procedure: Yang, the male principle, is represented by the left (hand) and Yin, the female element, is represented by the right (hand). Thus the supposition existed that the left pulse, i.e., that of Yang, indicated the diseases of men, while the right pulse, i.e., that of Yin, indicated the diseases of women. However, since both Yang and Yin are represented in both sexes, it was necessary to consult the pulses of both hands in order to make a complete diagnosis.
81. See translation, chapter 19.

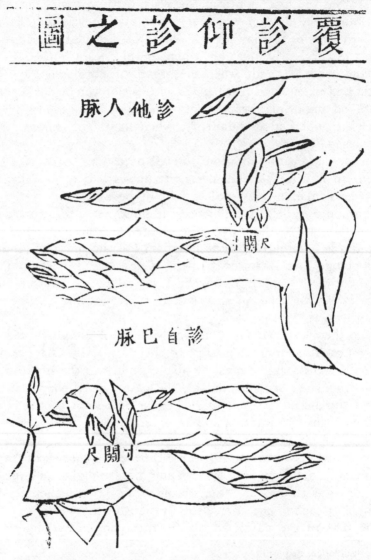

Fig. 14. The lower drawing shows how a physician feels his own pulse in order to compare it with the patient's pulse, as shown in the upper drawing. The three pulses are indicated on each wrist.

From: *T'u Chu Mo Chüeh*, by Chang Shih-hsien of the Ming period, published in 1510

that he must be able to judge the state of the disease—its cause and its duration, whether it was chronic or acute, whether it would result in death or in recovery—by the volume, strength, weakness, regularity or interruptions of the four main varieties of pulse beats. These four principal pulses are explained by Dr. K. Chimin Wong as: "*Fu* (浮) superficial, a light flowing pulse like a piece of wood floating on water; *Ch'en* (沉) deep, a deeply impressed pulse like a stone thrown into water; *Ch'ih* (遲) slow, a pulse with three beats to one cycle of respiration; and *Shu* (數) quick, a pulse with six beats to one cycle of respiration."[82] In addition to these main types there were a number of variations, many of which can be found in the chapters of the *Nei Ching* that deal with the pulse.[83]

The method that was supposed to make it possible to cope with the enormous task of palpation instructed the physician to lay a finger on each of the three sections of the pulse, each of which had a specific name; the one closest to the hand was called *tsun* (寸) or "inch," the one further up on the arm was called *ch'ih* (尺) or "cubit," and the one between the "inch" and the "cubit" pulses was called *kuan* (關) or "bar." The relationship between the internal and external pulses and the various organs as extracted from the *Nei Ching* is as follows:[84]

	Right Wrist	Left Wrist
"Inch" (寸)	lungs thoracic organs	heart mediastinal viscera
"Bar" (關)	stomach spleen	liver diaphragm
"Cubit" (尺)	kidney abdomen	kidney abdomen (small intestine)

The physician was instructed to take as norm of the pulse beats one expiration and one inspiration of his own, during which time the normal pulse should pulsate four times. The respiration of the patient was also of significance; and while taking the pulse, it was the physician's duty to watch the relationship between the number

82. Wong and Wu, *History of Chinese Medicine*, p. 42.
83. See translation, chapter 18.
84. See translation, chapter 17.

男左推三關六腑圖

女右推三關六腑圖

Illustration demonstrating how palpation should be applied to a man at his left wrist.

From Hsiao Erh T'ui Na Kuang I, a compilation of earlier writings on children's diseases, published in 1898.

Illustration demonstrating how palpation should be applied to a woman at her right wrist.

of pulse beats and the number of inspirations and exhalations of the patient and also whether his breathing was rough or smooth, light or heavy.[85]

As mentioned above, the pulse served not only for the purposes of diagnosis but also of prognosis. For this dual purpose the physician used additional methods of examination. These are summed up in chapter five: "Those who are experts in examining patients judge their general appearance; they feel the pulse and distinguish whether it is Yin or Yang that causes the disease. If the appearance changes from clear to turbid then the location of the disease is revealed. Coughing and short-windedness should be watched carefully; one should listen to the sounds and the notes and then the location of the affliction will become apparent."

In addition to these points, interrogation as to dreams and their interpretation played an important part in a complete examination.[86] The examination of the appearance, i.e., of the colors of the various parts of the body, was carried out according to the fixed system of correlations between colors and viscera, rather than according to actually observable phenomena. In chapter ten of the *Nei Ching* we find a number of combinations of certain colors and certain viscera denoting health and others denoting sickness and death. In chapter 17 we come upon minute descriptions as to how the combined examination of the pulse and the colors (complexion) yields diagnosis. The following sentence may serve as an illustration: "When the pulses of the liver and the kidneys coincide and the related colors are azure and red, the corresponding disease has destructive and injurious power."

After the location of the disease or the affected organ was known to the physician, he was able—by means of the fixed relationships—to determine the cause of the disease and also to prevent aggravating complications. Among the major causes of disease were thought to be the winds (風), which were held to disturb the harmony of Yin and Yang within the body. Thus when the patient suffered from an ailment of the liver, throat, or neck, it was held to be caused by the east wind; the ailments of the heart, chest and ribs were caused by the south wind; the west wind caused ailments of the lungs,

85. See translation, chapter 19.
86. See translation, chapter 17.

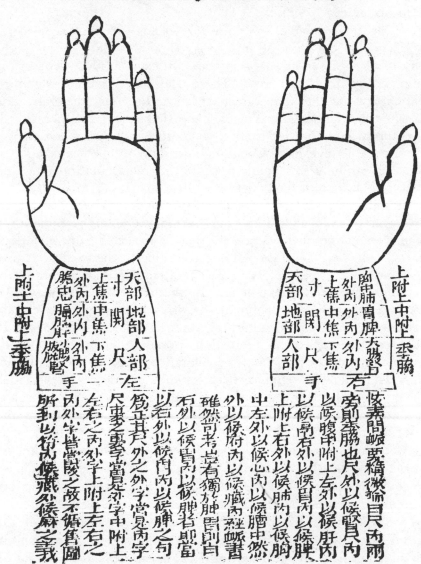

FIG. 16. DIAGRAM SHOWING THE ARRANGEMENT OF THE PULSES OF THE VISCERA
AND THE BOWELS

Reproduced from *The Golden Mirror*, an encyclopedia, containing the early medical writings of the Han dynasty (206 B.C.–220 A.D.), compiled under the edict of the emperor K'ang Hsi (1661–1722 A.D.).

shoulders, and back; and the north wind brought diseases of the kidneys, loins, and thighs. These four winds were believed to arise during particular seasons. But in addition to producing the winds, the seasons themselves produced certain diseases, which, if not checked in time, would recur or become aggravated during the following season.[87] Another cause of disease was of more general nature and could occur any time and affect any organ. It was described as "evil" or "noxious air" (邪 氣), was diagnosed by the usual means, and has frequently attributed to bad habits of living and infractions of the rules of the Tao.

DISEASES OF THE NEI CHING

It is logical that the concept of disease should have been based upon, and should be equally vague as, the physiological and anatomical concepts discussed above. The idea of a disease entity as it is known to Western medicine did not exist in ancient Chinese medical thought. And even symptomatology, although it was greatly stressed as an aid to the highly subtilized art of diagnosis, suffered from a general indefiniteness, for it too was forced into the realm of concordances.

The analysis of the diseases that are mentioned in the *Nei Ching* is extremely difficult. Even today when the ideographs representing the various ailments are translated into English with modern medical terms, we usually find that each ideograph has various meanings which are narrowed down only by the addition of a second ideograph with a restricting meaning. This fact might be illustrated in the following way:

(瘋) fêng: Paralysis. Leprosy. Insanity

(瘋 子): a maniac

(瘋 病): paralysis

(痲 瘋): leprosy

Since in connection with this ideograph, as well as in the majority of instances, the second, defining ideograph is absent in the *Nei Ching*, it is, of course, impossible to know which of these three kinds of disease was in the author's mind. Moreover, it is imperative to avoid the use of modern medical terms in a translation of this nature, for it is highly doubtful if any knowledge of an exact definition of diseases existed at the time when the *Nei Ching* was composed.

87. See translation, chapter 4.

As was mentioned in previous sections, the majority of ailments were chiefly attributed to the following causes: a dyscrasia of the five elements, i.e., a lack of balance between Yin and Yang, brought about either by the seasons directly or by the weather conditions peculiar to each season, or by infringements against the Tao. These ailments were generally called "injuries of the heart," "injuries of the lungs," etc., and were not designated by any specific terms. As a rule these injuries also extended to those organs and extremities which, according to the general concordances, were held to be subsidiary to the viscera. In addition to this general injury of the viscera, there is mentioned another, slightly more specific affliction, that of "numbness" (痺), which can befall all the viscera. This numbness, which was attributed to obstructions in the flow of blood, is diagnosed and described as follows.

"When the pulse has a red appearance and there is an obstinate cough, the examiner says that there is amassed air within (the heart) and it is dangerous to eat at this particular time. This disease is known as 'numbness of the heart.' It is contracted through external evil influences, causing anxiety and emptying the heart while the evil influences follow into it."[88]

Since, in keeping with the *Nei Ching*'s theory, longevity and health were identical, the process of aging was itself held to be a sign of disease and is described accordingly:

"When man grows old, his bones become dry and brittle like straw; his flesh sags and there is much gas within the thorax, resulting in laboured breathing. When he then cannot ease nature, he develops pains within his body. Then the top of his shoulders and the nape of his neck are contracted, his body burns with fever and his bones are stripped (of the flesh). This will become visible by the (pulse of the) spleen."[89]

The numbness mentioned above also occurs in connection with a group of diseases that are apparently of the nature of mental disturbances and are caused by five harmful emanations affecting Yin and Yang. The four other disturbances are wildness (狂), insanity (巔), loss of speech (瘖), and anger (怒).[90] Insanity, however, can

88. See translation, chapter 10.
89. See translation, chapter 19.
90. See translation, chapter 23.

also be produced by a special kind of air and appears in the following group of afflictions:

> Wind causes chills and fevers.
> Overwork causes exhaustion of the diaphragm.
> Oppressive airs cause insanity (madness 癲).
> Abundant winds cause ulcers (疽).[91]

Neither the form in which insanity manifests itself nor the nature of the ulcers is described in any detail.

The only diseases that are explained in a somewhat more circumstantial manner are a number of fevers, and of these "the injury of the cold" (傷 寒) receives the greatest attention. The ideographs for this injury of the cold stand in modern terminology for typhoid fever; but in ancient Chinese medicine they were used to designate many kinds of feverish illnesses, possibly of the nature of typhoid fever, but held to be caused by wind, actual injuries of the cold, or humid heat. The injury of the cold is described in chapter thirty-one:

"On the first day the injury of the cold is received by the great Yang. Therefore the head and the neck are in pain; the waist and the back become rigid. On the second day the region of the 'sunlight' receives the disease. The 'sunlight' controls the flesh, its pulse supports the nose and is connected with the eyes. Thus when the body is hot (feverish), the eyes ache, the nose is dry and the patient finds it impossible to rest. On the third day the region of the lesser Yang receives the disease. The region of the lesser Yang controls the gall bladder. Its pulse follows the flanks and is connected with the ears. Thus the ribs and the chest are in pain and the ears turn deaf. Now the three regions of Yang and the arteries have received the disease; however, it has not yet entered the viscera and therefore one can produce perspiration and terminate it."

This description continues until, on the sixth day, all parts of the body are affected by the disease. If at that time both the blood and the vital substances cease to move about, death follows. If, however, the patient remains alive after the crisis of the sixth day, there will be gradual improvement, during which the organs recover in the same order in which they were affected, so that, on the twelfth day, all symptoms of the disease disappear.

The next of these feverish diseases described by the *Nei Ching*

91. See translation, chapter 17.

is the "hot illness" (熱 病), which is mentioned in chapter thirty-two. The hot illness affects the five viscera individually and produces different effects in each of them:

"When the hot illness is located in the liver, first the urine turns yellow, then the stomach is in pain; the patient wishes to lie down and his body is hot (feverish). The elements of the heat conflict within the body and cause delirious speech and sudden starts during the sleep; the ribs and flanks are full of pain, the hands and feet are restless and the patient cannot lie down peacefully."

This is followed by a description of the hot illness as it affects the heart, the spleen, the lungs, and the kidneys.

Although the reports on the various pictures presented by the hot illness could be the result of actual observation, the description of the symptoms is again the result of the usual schematization:

"The symptoms of the sickness of the heat, when it is located in the liver, are that the left side of the jaw first turns red. The symptoms of the hot sickness, when it is located in the heart, are that the complexion first turns red. The symptoms of the hot sickness, when it is located in the spleen, are that the nose first turns red. The symptoms of the hot sickness, when it is located in the lungs, are that the right side of the jaw first turns red. The symptoms of the hot sickness, when it is located in the kidneys, are that the chin first turns red."[92]

Other fevers which belong to this group but are mentioned only in a cursory manner are the "wind within" (中 風), the "humid warmth"(濕 溫), and the "warm illness" (溫 病).[93]

Another fever which is not part of the group just discussed is the remittent or intermittent fever that occurs in fall and is usually held to be caused by an injury of the cold contracted during summer, or by insufficient perspiration during summer.[94] Although, as was pointed out above, it is dangerous to infer the existence of diseases as we know them now, there is some possibility that this intermittent fever may have been a form of malaria. The great emphasis that is put upon the spleen and its function throughout the *Nei Ching* may serve to substantiate this supposition. It is possible that disproportionate importance was given to the spleen by the early Chinese physicians, since they frequently saw it enlarged because of malarial inflammation.

92. See translation, chapter 32.
93. See translation, chapter 33.
94. See translation, chapter 4.

THERAPEUTIC CONCEPTS OF THE NEI CHING

In keeping with its insistence on maintaining the number five system in all aspects, the *Nei Ching* lists five methods of treatment: "The first method cures the spirit; the second gives knowledge on how to nourish the body; the third teaches the true effects of medicines; the fourth explains acupuncture and the use of the small and the large needle; the fifth gives instruction on how to examine and to treat the bowels and the viscera, the blood and the breath."[95] These methods are described as having developed one after the other to meet the gradually increasing demand for medical help.

The first method, the cure of the spirit, is representative of the closeness between Chinese religious and medical thinking and exemplifies their common base of universalism. The treatment of the spirit consisted in guiding towards Tao those persons who by infringement "of the basic rules of the universe [had] severed their own roots and ruined their true selves." For it was said that "those who disobey the laws of Heaven and Earth have a lifetime of calamities, while those who follow the laws remain free from dangerous illness."[96] Obedience towards the laws of heaven and earth is what Dr. Morse calls "spiritual alchemy,"[97] and it is practiced in a modest and retiring way of life, in the avoidance of all excesses, and in being an example to others in one's true devotion.

We read that in olden times, because of the simple mode of living of the ancients, diseases were few and mild and invocation of the gods was sufficient to cure the spirit, which in turn brought about the cure of the body.[98] Moreover, the ancients were reputed to have followed Tao and the laws of the seasons under the guidance of their sages, who were credited with the realization of the value of education in the prevention of disease, and of whom it was said: "The ancient sages did not treat those who were already ill; they instructed those who were not ill."[99]

But with the end of this tranquil era, which is pictured as being too primitive to admit evil influences, man became more violent, and therefore more vulnerable to noxious influences. "Evil influ-

95. See translation, chapter 25.
96. See translation, chapter 2.
97. Morse, *Chinese Medicine*, p. 24.
98. See translation, chapter 13.
99. See translation, chapter 2.

ences strike from early morning until late at night; they injure the
five viscera, the bones and the marrow within the body, and externally they injure the mind and reduce its intelligence and they
also injure the muscles and the flesh.   Hence the minor illnesses
are bound to become grave and the serious diseases are bound to
result in death.   Therefore the invocation of the gods is no longer
the way to cure."[100]

Thus it became necessary to develop methods of diagnosis—the
study of the pulse and the complexion—and to invent new cures.
As a result, the second method of treatment, that of dietetics, came
into being.   But the application of dietetics was not based upon the
unbiased examination of food; it too was founded on the theory of
cosmogony, the five elements and the concordances based thereon.
The *Nei Ching* states that "each of the diseases of the four seasons
and the five viscera reacts to that of the five flavors to which they
[the seasons and the viscera] correspond."[101]

The five flavors—pungent, sour, sweet, bitter, and salty—have
dispersing, gathering, retarding, strengthening, and softening effects.
But the flavors have these basic tendencies only in connection with
their related viscera;[102] in connection with the other viscera, their
tendencies change.   In chapter 22 the *Nei Ching* gives many examples that indicate the proper use of the five flavors in relation to
all viscera.   For those cases where a choice of flavors seems open
to the physician, the text explains the effect of the various flavors
upon the affected organ in order to indicate to the physician which
flavor he has to choose to achieve the desired effect.   The following
selections may illustrate the system: "The liver has a tendency to
disintegrate—pungent food dispels this tendency.   One uses pungent
food in order to supplement the functions of the liver, and sour food
in order to drain it.   The heart has a tendency to weaken—salty
food makes the heart pliable.   One uses salty food to strengthen the
heart, and sweet food to drain it."

The five flavors are represented in five kinds of nourishment, each
of which has a specific function:

1. *The medicines*, which attack the evil influences.   Wang Ping,
the commentator of the *Nei Ching*, explains these to consist of metal,

100. See translation, chapter 13.
101. See translation, chapter 22.
102. See chart of Main Concordances.

jade, earth, stones, grasses, wood, vegetables, fruit (berries, nuts)
insects (reptiles), fish, birds, and wild animals, while the text of the
Nei Ching itself mentions only roots, stalks, the topmost branches
of thyme, herbs in general, and soups, clear liquids, lees of wine,
and sweet wines which were prepared from the five kinds of grain.
The recipes for the preparation of these medicinal drinks are very
simple, as can be seen in the instruction for the preparation of a
rice gruel: "One must use paddy rice and steam it. The stalks of
the rice serve as fire wood. When the steaming of the rice is completed, the rice (gruel) is very strong."[103]   The medicines were held
to be effective because they represented a mixture of the essences
of heaven and earth, the exalted and the base substances, in proper
proportions. It was also considered important to cut the plants
during the season having the closest affinity to the affected organ.

2. *The five grains*, which act as nourishment. They are wheat,
glutinous millet, millet, rice, and beans.

3. *The five tree-fruits*, which serve to augment the nourishment.
They are peaches, plums, apricots, chestnuts, and dates.

4. *The five domestic animals*, which contribute additional nutri-
tional benefit. They are fowl, sheep, beef, horses and pigs.

5. *The five vegetables*, which complete nourishment. They are
mallows, coarse greens, scallions, onions, and leeks.[104]

The five flavors are effective not only upon the five viscera but
upon all parts of the body that are connected with the viscera.
Thus we read: "If people pay attention to the five flavors and blend
them well, their bones will remain straight, their muscles will remain
tender and young, breath and blood will circulate freely, the pores
will be fine in texture, and consequently breath and bones will be
filled with the essence of life."[105]

While in chapter thirteen the various methods of treatment are
described as having evolved successively, chapter twelve states that
the development of the different cures resulted from the various
geographical conditions under which the people lived. The four
points of the compass and the region of the center are held to produce
anthropological differences and, consequently, susceptibility to different diseases in man; and these, in turn, can be cured only by that

103. See translation, chapter 22.
104. See translation, chapter 14.
105. See translation, chapter 3.

method which is supposed to be connected specifically with each particular region. The five cures employed in this chapter differ from those mentioned earlier, for here the study of nutrition and the related laws of the flavors become superfluous as healing methods, since nutrition and living habits are determined by geographical and climatic necessity.

The system of therapy evolved from this chapter works in the following manner: The people of the East live near the ocean and eat much fish and salt. Fish and seafood are thought to cause an "internal burning," salt to injure the blood. These factors cause a dark complexion and a propensity towards ulcers, which must be treated with acupuncture by means of a needle of flint.

The people of the West live in dwellings of stone, their fields are fertile and their food good and varied. Because their land is hilly and exposed to the wind and their clothes made of coarse wool or matting, their bodies are robust and healthy and impervious to external diseases. Their internal diseases must be cured with (poison) medicine.[106]

The people of the North live in mountainous regions; their food consists mainly of milk products. They are exposed to cold winds and frost and hence suffer from many diseases which must be treated with moxa.

The people of the South live in regions which are fertile through an abundance of sun and dew (although their waters are beneath the earth and the soil is deficient). They live on sour food and curd, and they suffer from contracted muscles and numbness and should be treated with acupuncture by means of the nine fine needles.

The people who inhabit the Center live on level, fertile ground and are able to obtain a varied diet without great exertion. Yet, they too are attacked by disease, mainly by complete paralysis, chills and fevers. The treatment prescribed for the people of the Center consists of massage, breathing exercises, and exercises of the extremities.

106. The nature of these poison medicines is not disclosed in the text of the *Nei Ching*. However, since the commentator, Wang Ping, mentions reptiles, insects, and other animals as belonging to the materia medica of the *Nei Ching*, it can be presumed that the poison medicines here referred to are identical with the "five poisons" that are generally enumerated in works dealing with the Chinese materia medica. They are extracted from the five poisonous "reptiles" (creatures), the viper, the scorpion, the centipede, the toad, and the lizard.

Of these five methods of healing, the one by means of medicines has been discussed above. The practice of massage has been employed by Western medicine and needs no further explanation. The cures connected with the East and the South are variations of acupuncture, one of the most widely applied treatments in Chinese medical history. Acupuncture and moxa, the method applied to the people of the North, will be discussed in the next section.

It is interesting to note that in contrast to the subtilized methods of diagnosis—the observation of the complexion and, chiefly, the study of the pulse—therapeutic measures, with the exception of acupuncture, receive very little detailed description. This leads to the impression that diagnosis and therapy were not sharply divided and that the physician would know which treatment he was to apply once the diagnosis was made. The theory that the diagnosis was of prime importance and that the physician would be familiar with the practical application of therapeutic measures finds support in sentences like this: "The most important requirement of the art of healing is that no mistakes or neglect occur. There should be no doubt or confusion as to the application of the term of 'complexion and pulse.' These are the maxims of the art of healing."[107]

A medical practice that was based almost entirely upon the complicated method of palpation, coupled with the observation of external changes, necessarily required particularly conscientious and alert physicians to produce tangible results. This was realized by the authors of the *Nei Ching*, who repeatedly warned that "poor medical workmanship is neglectful and careless and must therefore be combatted, because a disease that is not completely cured can easily breed new disease or there can be a recurrence of the old disease,"[108] and "illness is comparable to the root; good medical work is comparable to the topmost branch; if the root is not reached, the evil influences cannot be subjugated."[109] But the physician was not only cautioned to prevent relapses or an aggravation of the disease; he was also made conscious that the greatest medical art was the diagnosis of a disease at the stage of its inception. "The superior physician helps before the early budding of the disease. The inferior physician begins to help when the disease has already

107. See translation, chapter 13.
108. See translation, chapter 13.
109. See translation, chapter 14.

developed; he helps when destruction has already set in.   And since his help comes when the disease has already developed, it is said of him that he is ignorant."[110]

In order to guide the physician in his search for symptoms, the *Nei Ching* furnishes a definition of health which is expressed in the rhythm of breathing in relation to the pulse beats.   Since the physician uses his own respiration as a norm when taking the pulse of a patient, it is imperative that his own health and hence his respiration be in perfect order.   Thus it is said: "Those who are habitually without disease help to train and to adjust those who are sick, for those who treat should be free from illness.   They train the patient to adjust his breathing, and in order to train the patient, they act as examples."[111]

The possible use of surgery is mentioned twice; at one occasion it is considered as a last resort when all other remedies fail, at another instance in connection with the treatment of ulcers, where a recourse to cutting and scooping out of exposed and spoiled particles is suggested but accompanied by a warning against hasty use.   In general, however, the *Nei Ching* prefers to cure disease by bringing into harmony the disturbed elemental cosmic forces by means of education and the more orthodox methods of treatment: the physician should criticize and correct the faults in the patient's mode of life; he should restore the body by "opening the anus so that the bowels can be cleaned, and that the secretions come at the proper time and serve the viscera, which belong to the principle of Yang."[112]

ACUPUNCTURE AND MOXIBUSTION

The domination of Chinese medicine by the theories of cosmogony finds its strongest expression in the two ancient methods of healing: acupuncture and moxibustion.   At the time when the *Nei Ching* was composed both these treatments must have been well known, for, although there are numerous references containing indications for their use, there is very little information concerning the method of their application and no reference at all containing those basic instructions which would have been inevitably necessary, had the

110. See translation, chapter 26.
111. See translation, chapter 18.
112. See translation, chapter 14.

Nei Ching itself introduced these methods. Hence one must have recourse to additional works on the subject in order to receive a complete picture of these important means of treatment, which have remained in use up to the present day.[113]

The application of acupuncture, which is also called "needling," consists of the insertion of needles of various materials and shapes into particular points of the body. The *Nei Ching* mentions the use of nine kinds of needles,[114] which are explained by Dr. K. Chimin Wong to be "arrow-headed, blunt, puncturing, spear-pointed, ensiform, round, capillary, long, and great [big]."[115] Their length varies from 3 to 24 cm.[116] In ancient times these needles were made of flint, later of gold, silver, steel, or iron. Dr. Nakayama mentions that the selection of the metal was conditioned by the individual case in which the needles were to be employed. "A Chinese theory attributes to the yellow metals [Yang], gold, copper, etc., a stimulating, vivifying power; and to the white metals [Yin], silver, chrome, zinc, etc., a calming, dispersing power."[117]

The points of acupuncture are distributed all over the body, the head and the extremities, and represent strategic points along the twelve channels or main ducts. According to Dr. Morse these channels "are what might be designated as the 'outside' control of the blood vessels which are themselves 'internal' and which more intimately connect the organs and viscera. The channels are supposed to be deeply set in the muscles and not in *direct connection* with the blood vessels."[118]

As may be remembered from the earlier discussion of the Chinese theory of angiology and splanchnology, there exists a fixed interrelationship between various organs of the body: the liver is connected with the gall bladder and the ligaments; the heart is connected with the small intestines and the arteries; the spleen is connected

113. For the discussion of the origin and the theory of acupuncture and moxa I have used Hsieh, "A Review of Ancient Chinese Anatomy," pp. 117-121; Nakayama, *Acupuncture et Médecine chinoise*; Wong and Wu, *History of Chinese Medicine*, pp. 28-29; Morse, *Chinese Medicine*, pp. 137-161; P. Dabry, *La Médecine chez les Chinois*, ouvrage corrigé et précédé d'une préface par M. J. Léon Soubeiran (Paris, 1863), pp. 421-497; G. Soulié de Morant, *Précis de la vraie acuponcture chinoise* (Paris, 1935).

114. See translation, chapter 12.

115. Wong and Wu, *History of Chinese Medicine*, p. 29.

116. Morse, *Chinese Medicine*, p. 137.

117. Nakayama, *Acupuncture et Médecine chinoise*, p. 48 (1).

118. Morse, *Chinese Medicine*, p. 137.

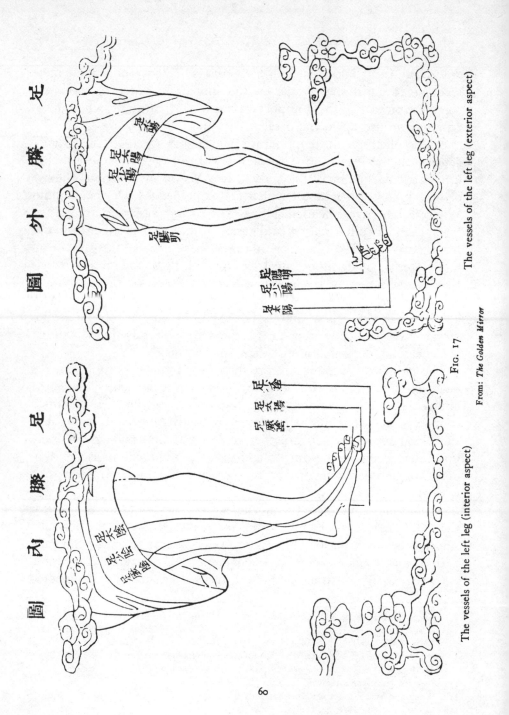

足 膝 外 圖

足 膝 內 圖

足少陽膽

足太陽膀胱

足陽明

足陽明
足少陽
足太陽

足太陰

足少陰

足厥陰

足厥陰
足太陰
足少陰

The vessels of the left leg (interior aspect)

The vessels of the left leg (exterior aspect)

Fig. 17

From: *The Golden Mirror*

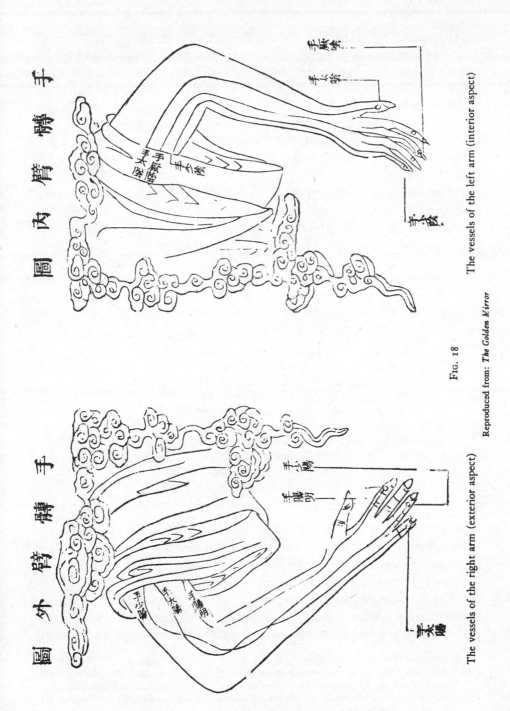

手 臂 臑 內 圖

手厥陰心包絡
手太陰肺

手少陰心

手太陰
手少陰

手厥陰

The vessels of the left arm (interior aspect)

手 臑 臂 外 圖

手陽明
手太陽

手太陽
手陽明
手少陽

手少陽

The vessels of the right arm (exterior aspect)

FIG. 18

Reproduced from: *The Golden Mirror*

with the stomach and the muscles; the lungs are connected with the large intestines and the skin; the kidneys are connected with the three burning spaces, the bladder and the bones.[119]   The connections themselves are created by the supposed existence of the system of ducts, the function of which is to cause circulation of the blood and air, to moisten the bones and ligaments and to lubricate the joints.

The twelve main ducts come in pairs and are arranged symmetrically on the left and the right side of the body.   Six ducts or vessels belong to the principle of Yin and six to the principle Yang so that two vessels are attributed to each of the three subdivisions of Yin and Yang.   The names of the vessels indicate their respective affinities to the elemental forces and to particular organs of the body.[120]   Dr. E. T. Hsieh enumerates their routes as follows.[121]

1. From the middle burning space to the tip of the thumb.
2. From the tip of the thumb and the small finger to the large intestine.
3. From the middle of the nose to the middle of the foot.
4. From the great toe to the lower part of the tongue.
5. From the heart to the inside of the little finger.
6. From the little finger to the small intestine.
7. From the inner corner of the eye to the little toe.
8. From the little toe to the root of the tongue.
9. From the middle of the stomach to the tip of the middle finger.
10. From the tip of the little finger to the three burning spaces.
11. From the outer angles of the eyes to the little toes.
12. From the hairy spots on the big toes to the vertex of the head.

As mentioned above, these channels are deeply imbedded in the muscles; at three hundred and sixty-five points, however, they emerge to the surface and thus present the points for needling.   The number three hundred sixty-five is significant, for it parallels the days of the year as well as the muscular junctions of the body.

The confidence in the therapeutic value of acupuncture is closely connected with the belief in the forces that created the world and whose interaction causes the balance within the universe and within

119. See main chart of concordances.
120. The names are "hand great female [great Yin 太 陰] lung vessels," "hand great male [great Yang 太 陽] small intestine vessels," etc.   Six pairs of ducts are "hand vessels," and six pairs are "foot vessels," depending on whether the vessels originate from or end in the hands or in the feet.
121. Hsieh, "A Review of Ancient Chinese Anatomy," p. 118.

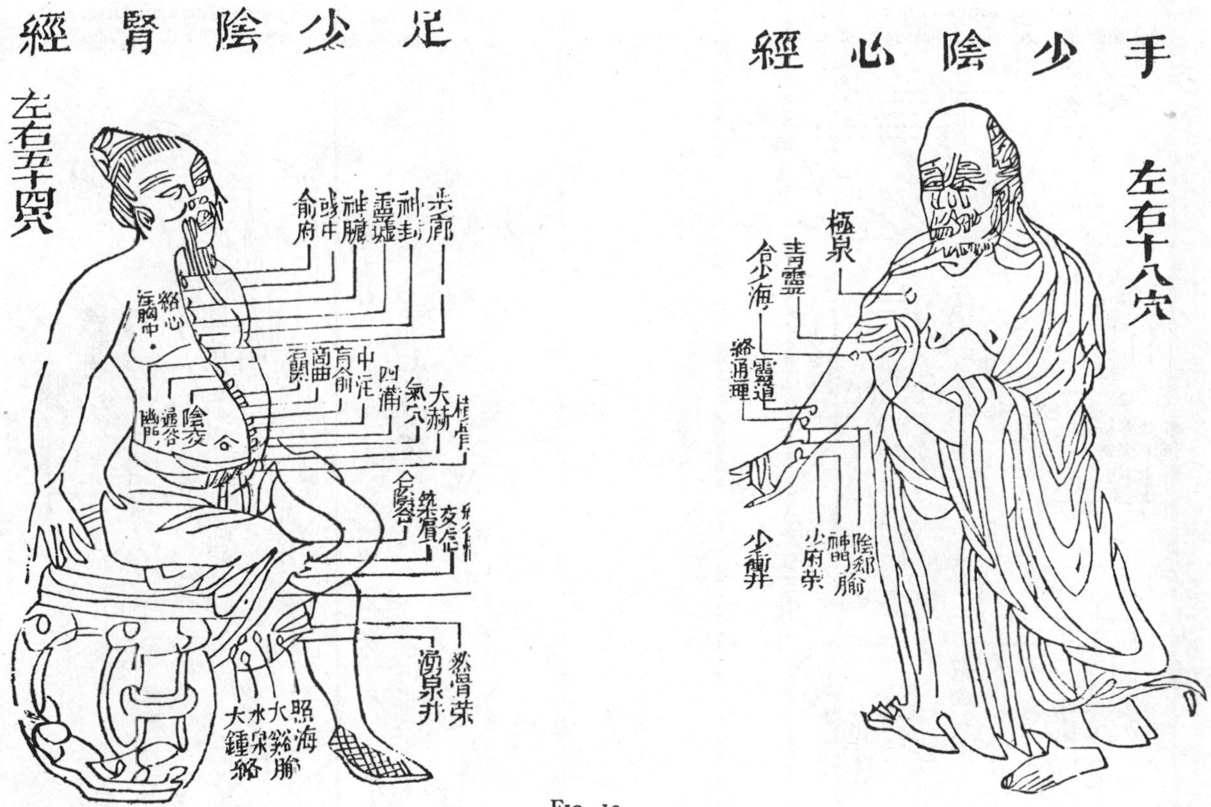

手少陰心經

The heart vessel of the lesser Yin showing
9 acupuncture spots

足少陰腎經

The kidney vessel of the lesser Yin showing
29 acupuncture spots

FIG. 19

From: *Ling Shu Su Wên Chieh Yao*

63

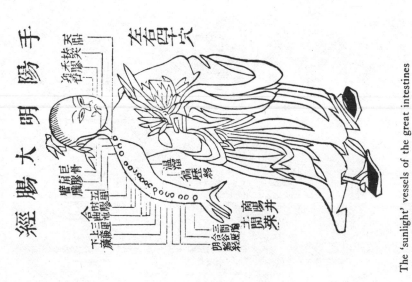

The 'sunlight' vessels of the great intestines
showing 20 acupuncture spots

The 'sunlight' vessel of the stomach showing
48 acupuncture spots

FIG. 20

From: *Ling Shu Su Wên Chieh Yao*

the body. These forces, Yin and Yang, are theoretically supposed to balance each other completely but are, in reality, in a constant state of conquest and defeat, of ebb and flow, as it is expressed in nature in the change from day to night. Within the body, too, the distribution of the two elemental forces is uneven, as was shown in the earlier section dealing with Yin and Yang in the *Nei Ching*. The complicated relationship of the dual power with the various parts of the body can function smoothly only if the flux of Yin and Yang is uninterrupted. When there is stagnation in certain parts of the body and hence a deficiency in others, the result is disease. The twelve ducts are the supposed carriers of the two cosmic forces, and if stagnation occurs it takes place within these channels. It is thought that by puncturing the channels at those points which are connected with the diseased organ, the evil air that caused the stagnation is forced to escape and circulation can set in again. Dr. Nakayama explains the theory of acupuncture as follows: "The needles, whether of gold, silver, iron, chrome or other metal, are, from the Yin-Yang point of view of the elements, charged with the activity of Yin . . . that is to say, dilatory, centrifugal, relaxing, calming, by the system [of the ducts]. They restore all cells and organs by giving the stimulus of Yin. Consequently, acupuncture is primarily recommended for all excess of Yang. But through the equilibrium of Yang, which it gives to the organism, it restores the energy of Yin and indirectly gives favorable results in maladies of Yin, in addition to its direct stimulating action on Yin."[122]

Moxa, or moxibustion, has a purpose similar to acupuncture, that is, to bring into proper balance the flow of Yin and Yang. Dr. Nakayama has expressed it as follows: "Moxibustion (ignipuncture) which is based on heat is therefore of the nature of Yang. It is very highly recommended in all diseases which are caused by the excess of Yin. Activity of the blood, production of albuminoids, congestion, etc., are all Yang by nature."[123]

The practice of moxibustion consists of the application to the skin of combustible cones of powdered leaves of Artemisia vulgaris. These cones are placed on particular spots and are ignited; they are extinguished only after they burn down to the skin and a blister is formed. There are separate charts for moxibustion which usually

122. Nakayama, *Acupuncture et Médecine chinoise*, p. 48.
123. *Ibid.*, p. 50.

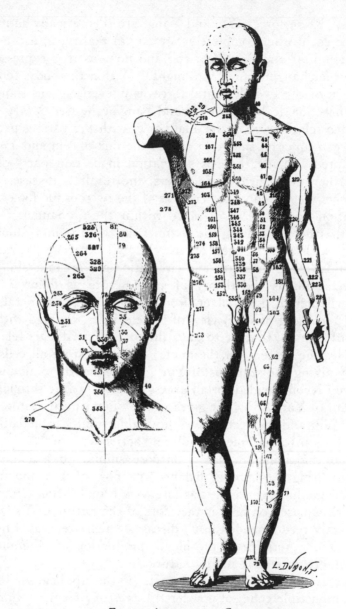

FIG. 21. ACUPUNCTURE CHART

Reproduced from: P. Dabry, *La Médecine chez les Chinois*, ouvrage corrigé et précédé d'une préface par
M. J. Léon Soubeiran. Paris, 1863

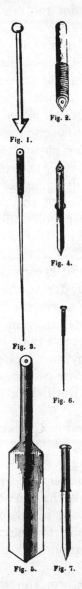

Fig. 3.

Fig. 1.

Fig. 4.

Fig. 3.

Fig. 6.

Fig. 5.   Fig. 7.

FIG. 22. ACUPUNCTURE NEEDLES

Reproduced from: P. Dabry, *La Médecine chez les Chinois*

show a symmetric pattern, for the most part applied to the back; but moxa can sometimes also be applied to the acupuncture points after the needle has been withdrawn.

Although the *Nei Ching* does not discuss the theoretical foundations for application of moxa and acupuncture nor teach the actual technique of their use, the treatise gives detailed instructions as to the proper times and indications when the two remedies should be applied. In order to find an auspicious moment for the application of acupuncture and moxa, the physician must establish the position of the heavenly bodies, their relation to the prevailing season, and the weather conditions resulting therefrom. Since acupuncture is applied to remove stagnation of the flow of Yin and Yang, it is necessary to perform this operation under climatic conditions that in themselves favor the flow of the two elements. In warm and sunny weather, during the period while the moon is waxing or full, the movement of man's blood and breath is held to be in the best condition; while in cold weather, during the period of the waning moon, man's blood is held to have a tendency to coagulate and his breath to become weakened. Smooth movement of breath and blood present the most advantageous conditions for the flow of Yin and Yang. Stagnation can be caused by two factors: a plethora of Yang or a deficiency of Yin. Either state can occur independently, or one can be the cause of the other. Both these failings are indicated by the pulse beats.

The *Nei Ching* teaches that acupuncture applied to a plethora of Yang has a "draining" effect, while in the case of a deficiency of Yin, acupuncture supplements vigor. Both draining and supplementing must be performed under proper atmospheric conditions, which are described in chapter 26. "At the time of the new moon one should not drain and when the moon is full one should not supplement. When the moon is empty to the rim one cannot heal diseases. Hence one should consult the weather and the seasons and adjust [the treatment] to them."

Having found the proper atmospheric conditions for his undertaking, the physician has to adjust his operation to the breathing of his patient. The needle must be inserted at the time of inhalation, then it is twisted around and extracted with the next exhalation. Although it seems self-evident, the *Nei Ching* emphasizes that during this process the hand of the practitioner must be calm and the action

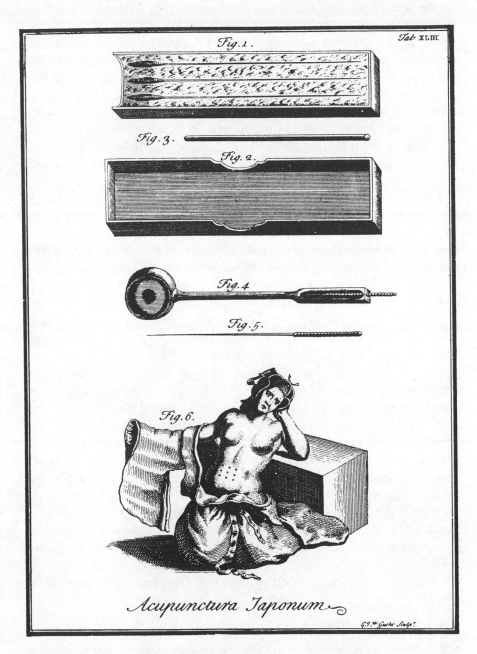

Acupunctura Japonum

FIG. 23

From: Engelbert Kaempfer's: *Histoire naturelle, civile, et ecclésiastique de l'empire du Japon*, La Haye, 1729

of the needle uniform in every performance.[124] Before the actual treatment with acupuncture or moxa begins, the physician is instructed to measure the thorax in order to be able to determine the approximate location of the viscera. The physician must also inform himself about the extent and the location of the various regions of Yin and Yang, for it is held that the contents of blood and air vary in each region and consequently also the substance that issues forth during the process of puncturing. "When one punctures the region of the 'sunlight' (陽 明) blood and air issue forth; when one punctures the region of the lesser Yang (少 陽)air and noxious blood issue forth . . . etc."[125] However, the substance that escapes from the various points of needling is considered important not so much because of its own consistency but rather because it is held to be the carrier for the evil influences that brought about the disease, and it is these evil influences which are caused to depart by the application of acupuncture.[126] Except for the chapter on the geographical origin of various medications, the *Nei Ching* does not contain any separate instructions as to the use of moxa; the indications for its application are the same as for needling, and it is not quite clear whether they are recommended as alternative remedies or whether they should be applied together.

As was mentioned at the beginning of this Introduction, the practice of orthodox Chinese medicine has continued to the present day without major changes ever since the *Huang Ti Nei Ching Su Wên* was composed. The taking of the pulse is still the most important means of diagnosis.[127] Medicines derived from the mineral, animal and vegetable kingdoms, though more numerous and more specific than described in the *Nei Ching*, are still applied according to the elemental principles that are the basis of Chinese cosmogony. And even the practice of acupuncture and moxibustion has survived, despite the fact that these treatments must be exceedingly painful to the patient. These treatments have survived not only in China where they were conceived but also in Japan, whither they migrated as a part of the medical art which the Japanese took over from

---

124. See translation, chapter 25.
125. See translation, chapter 24.
126. See translation, chapter 10.
127. Bernard E. Read, "Gleanings from Old Chinese Medicine," *Annals of Medical History*, VIII (1926), 16–19; see also Morse, *Chinese Medicine*, p. 81; *et al.*

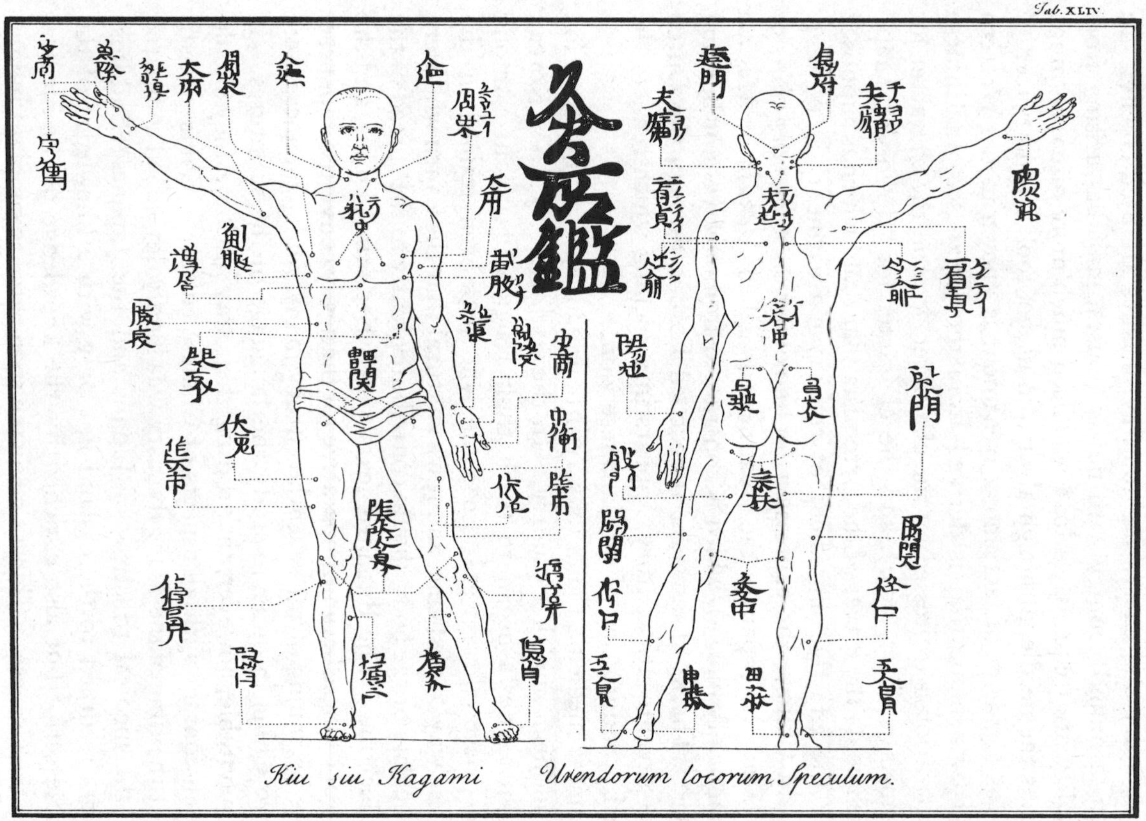

Tab. XLIV.

Kiu siu Kagami   *Unendorum locorum Speculum.*

FIG. 24. MOXIBUSTION CHART

From: Engelbert Kaempfer's: *Histoire naturelle, civile, et ecclésiastique de l'empire du Japon*, La Haye, 1729

71

China.   G. Soulié de Morant, in his preface to Dr. Nakayama's book
on acupuncture and Chinese medicine, states: "In Northern
China, a dry and enervating country, needles are used chiefly.   In
Japan, a humid country with flimsy houses, maladies arising from
humidity are frequent.   Moxa was used much more often; so much
so, that the needle, although always in usage, took second place."[128]
And, as a matter of fact, moxa treatment is known to the Western
world by a name that is derived from the Japanese.   In Chinese
cauterization is expressed by the character 灸 chiu, the character for
Artemisia is 艾 ai (ngai), and the character for "down" or "nap"
(which coats the leaves of the Artemisia plant and which is supposed
to be the effective ingredient of the moxa treatment) is 絨 jung.
Thus in Chinese the expression for moxibustion is ai jung chiu, or
just chiu.   In Japanese the treatment is called Mokusa or Mogusa
(phonetically mǫksa), which is contracted from moe kusa or burning
herb.[129]   The word moxa, as it reached Europe through the Dutch
in the seventeenth century, appears in a spelling which renders the
actual pronunciation of the Japanese word.

Chinese medicine found its way into Japan with the introduction
of Buddhism into that country.   In the sixth century A.D., Korean
Buddhist priests began to teach their religion in Japan.   Among
these priests there were also some who had been trained in the
Chinese way of medicine, and it was natural that these men who were
also healers of the body should contribute greatly to the spread of the
new doctrine.   The Buddhist texts were written in Chinese, and the
study of Chinese became imperative for the newly converted Japanese.
In the beginning of the seventh century many young Japanese were
sent to China in order to study the language of the scriptures.   It
was inevitable, however, that during their stay in China they should
come in contact with all aspects of Chinese culture.   Chinese medicine at the time of the T'ang dynasty was highly developed compared
with the medical practices of Japan, and the Japanese Buddhist
scholars returned to their island not only with a knowledge of the
Chinese script but also enriched by the knowledge of the medical
art of the Chinese.   Chinese medicine soon came to supplant indigenous Japanese practices, particularly after the study of the ideo-

128. Nakayama, *Acupuncture et Médecine Chinoise*, p. 12.
129. *The New English Dictionary* (Oxford, 1908), *s.v.* moxa; *Dictionnaire de la Langue française*,
    by Emile Littré (Paris, 1881), *s.v.* moxa.

graphs had made Chinese medical texts available to many Japanese. From then on—with slight modifications—Chinese medicine ruled supreme in Japan until, in the late sixteenth century, Portuguese priests and, in the seventeenth century, the physicians of the Dutch East India Company introduced European medicine.[130]

European medicine was adopted more quickly and extensively in Japan than in China. Numerous European medical works were translated into Japanese; for instance, abstracts from the works of Ambroise Paré were published as early as 1706.[131] And when, in 1884, the medical faculty of the University of Tokyo was founded, an edict was issued forbidding the teaching of the ancient methods altogether.[132] Nevertheless what has happened in Japan is similar to the course of medical history in China: the orthodox medical practices have continued to exist side by side with Western medicine. One reason for the continuance of orthodox medicine may lie in the fact that it was in both countries so closely connected with religion. In China medical theories are actually a part of the religion of Universalism. In Japan, Chinese medicine was, so to speak, a by-product of the conversion to Buddhism. But the other reason for the maintenance of these cumbersome and probably painful ways of treatment must be that they do possess a healing power, in spite of the condescension with which Westerners are apt to speak of pulse diagnosis and acupuncture and moxa treatments.

Some of the modern Japanese physicians, aware of the co-existence of their own Western medical techniques and the ancient practices, have been unable to close their eyes to the obvious effectiveness of acupuncture and moxa. In order to determine whether the treatments had actual curative powers, beyond a psychological effect, they have studied moxa and acupuncture by means of modern laboratory methods. Dr. Nakayama, the outstanding scientist of this group, has collected the following conclusions of some of his colleagues: "Dr. Hara, one of these scientists, after long studies pursued for years, has recently made available laboratory proofs that demonstrate that moxibustion increases the number of red

130. The history of the adoption of foreign medical practices by the Japanese is taken from Y. Fujikawa, *Japanese Medicine*, tr. from the German by John Ruhräh (Clio Medica, New York, 1934).
131. *Ibid.*, p. 79.
132. G. Soulié de Morant in Nakayama, *Acupuncture et Médecine chinoise*, p. 14.

corpuscles and hemoglobin.　The needles have a similar effect. . . .[133] Another insists on specific arterial congestion brought about by this method. . . .　Another scientist insists on the psychological efficacy. . . .　Another insists upon a particular arterial congestion, provoked by this method.　Another scientist proposes an entirely different hypothesis.　According to him, the efficacy of the method depends on a vigorous activation of the circulation by increase of arterial concentration, which would remove all pathological phenomena. . . . Another physician . . . concluded that the effect of moxibustion comes from an albuminoid produced during the burnings of moxa . . . on our skin. . . ."[134]

Dr. Nakayama's own conclusions were reached after the completion of a great number of clinical tests in which a vast variety of diseases had greatly improved after the application of either moxa or acupuncture.　He found that both remedies exert great influence upon the blood.　"A fact that seems unbelievable is that the blood is affected by moxibustion and acupuncture.　Immediately after the first treatment, it must be admitted, little difference can be noted. But through controlled moxibustion carried out for some length of time, the blood undergoes a materially important transformation. The needles produce [even] faster results."[135]　But while he appends case histories, charts and diagrams in support of his evidence, the essence of his discovery is contained in the following statement, applying the results of Western clinical research to the ancient Chinese theories of cosmogony which were the traditional basis for the remedy: "Since moxibustion represents a physical therapy of the nature of Yang, it should be used to cure all excess of Yin.　But moxibustion, being in fact a physical stimulus, also animates all physiological functions in a general way: metabolism, activity of the leucocytes, those of the nervous and psychic centers.　Insofar as physico-pharmaceutical stimulus is concerned, it has therefore an equally favorable and efficacious result in troubles of the nature of Yang."[136]

Dr. Nakayama's statement reflects the point of view and methodology of a modern physician combined with a firm belief in the

133. Dr. Hara's charts which prove his findings are contained in Dr. Nakayama's book.
134. Nakayama, *Acupuncture et Médecine chinoise*, p. 49.
135. *Ibid.*, p. 56.
136. Nakayama, *Acupuncture et Médecine chinoise*, p. 50.

validity of the system of Yin and Yang. Such attitudes, together with the popular appeal which the theory of Yin and Yang continues to enjoy, helps to explain why acupuncture and moxibustion have remained popular remedies for thousands of years. Nevertheless, it is startling to see that moxa, one of the oldest remedies in existence and mentioned in the most ancient Chinese medical treatise, was used in Hiroshima on August 6, 1945, and actually brought relief to one of the sufferers from the effects of the first atom bomb. In his epic story "Hiroshima"[137], John Hersey describes the fate of the people of that stricken city, and, especially, of six persons who had been at an approximate distance of two miles from the focus of the explosion. Four of these six people, like so many others who had survived the first impact of the bomb, fell ill from radiation sickness ten to fifteen days later. Mr. Hersey tells that "twenty-five to thirty days after the explosion, blood disorders appeared: gums bled, the white blood-cell count dropped sharply. . . . The two key symptoms, on which the doctors came to base their diagnosis, were fever and the lowered white-corpuscle count."[138]

One of the six specified survivors, the Reverend Tanimoto, a graduate in theology of Emory College, Atlanta, Georgia, who had been two miles away from the center of the explosion, took sick about two weeks later "with a general malaise, weariness and feverishness."[139] Since his health did not improve he sent for medical help, but the subsequent injections of Vitamin B 1 did little to better his state. After a few days, however, "a Buddhist priest with whom Mr. Tanimoto was acquainted called on him and suggested that moxibustion might give him relief; the priest showed the pastor how to give himself the ancient Japanese treatment, by setting fire to a twist of the stimulant herb moxa placed on the wrist pulse.[140] Mr. Tanimoto found that each moxa treatment temporarily reduced his fever one degree."[141] Dr. Nakayama's research on the effect of moxa upon the blood[142] makes one appreciate the instinctive wisdom which lay in the application of moxibustion in this case. It is pos-

137. John Hersey, "Hiroshima," *The New Yorker*, August 31, 1946.
138. *Ibid.*, p. 48.
139. *Ibid.*, p. 44.
140. It is unusual to apply moxa to the wrist pulse. The more common place for moxibustion is the region of the vertebra and the chest.
141. Hersey, "Hiroshima," p. 48.
142. Nakayama, *Acupuncture et Médecine chinoise*, pp. 56 ff.

sible that the treatment—had it been continued for an extended period—might have caused a quicker recovery than was achieved by the methods which were applied. But even the temporary relief caused by this ancient remedy is an indication of the great value contained within the universalistic medical system which found its first expression in the *Yellow Emperor's Canon of Internal Medicine*.

This repository of Chinese classical medical theory and practice still remains influential. It embodies the experience of an old and great people in wrestling with the problems of mortal ills and the preservation of human health. It indicates the closest possible integration between moral and physical conduct, and is therefore an early adumbration of the relationship between mental and physical states of health. As the basis of all subsequent medical writing in China and Japan, it affected the destinies of the peoples in a large part of the oriental world for thousands of years.

If the history of the *Yellow Emperor's Classic* is to be compared with that of the *Corpus Hippocraticum*, which originated at about the same time, a curious and somewhat contradictory development may be noted. The works of the Greek tradition were composed to serve as text-books for the practitioner, yet the practical value of their contents was superseded centuries ago. Apart from their significance for the medical historian, the value of these works has for centuries consisted in creating for the Western physician the moral and ethical concept of the ideal physician. On the other hand, it should be evident from the preceding discussion that China's earliest book concerned with the art of healing was never meant to be a mere text-book of medicine, but rather a treatise on the philosophy of health and disease; and yet it was taken over by the physician, not simply as a guide towards an ideal of life, but as a help for the actual practice of medicine.

It is not within the scope of this Introduction to make further comparison between the literary monuments of two such divergent traditions, but it is hoped that the modern Western doctor, whose spiritual ancestor is Hippocrates, and who today is trained in clinical and scientific research and the recognition of psychosomatic aspects of disease, will not fail to widen his horizon by discovering the philosophical wisdom of the *Yellow Emperor's Classic of Internal Medicine*.

APPENDIX I

Chapter 103 of the *Ssu-k'u Ch'üan-shu*[1] dealing with the *Huang Ti Su Wên*, 24 books

Commentary by Wang Ping of the T'ang Dynasty

ACCORDING to the "Treatise on the Canons and Literature"[2] the the *History of the Former Han Dynasty*[3] the *Huang Ti Nei Ching* consisted of only eighteen books and did not carry the (additional) title of "Su Wên." Chang Chi[4] of the later Han dynasty quoted this work in his *Treatise on Typhoid Fever* and began to call it Su Wên. In the Chin dynasty it was mentioned in the preface to the *Chia I Ching*[5] of Huang-fu Mi[6] that there were nine rolls of the "Classic of Acupuncture"[7] and nine rolls of "Simple Questions"[8] and that both of them were parts of the *Nei Ching*; (thus) its total number of books coincided with the eighteen fascicles mentioned in the *History of the Former Han Dynasty*. Thus we know that the name of Su Wên had originated at the time of the Han and Chin dynasties and was first recorded in the "Record of Books"[9] of the *Annals of the Sui Dynasty*.[10] But there were only eight rolls recorded in the "Record of Books" of the *Sui Annals*. And when Ch'üan Yüan-ch'i[11] made his commentary (upon the *Nei Ching*) the seventh (roll) had already been lost.

1. 四庫全書總目提要　*Collection of the Four Imperial Libraries* published under the authorization of the Chinese government in 1772 and completed in 1790 under Emperor Chien Lung. Edited by Yung Jung and others. Shanghai, The Commercial Press, Ltd., 1933.
2. 藝文志
3. *Han Shu.*
4. 張機. Commonly known as Chang Chung-ching 張仲景, the author of the famous *Treatise on Typhoid Fever*. His exact dates have not been established, but it is known that he held the office as mayor of Changsha in Hunan Province in 195 A.D.
5. 甲乙經　See footnote 6.
6. 皇甫謐, author of the *Chia I Ching*, flourished between 215 and 282 A.D. The book consists of 12 rolls and describes treatments by means of acupuncture and moxa.
7. 鍼經
8. 素問
9. 經籍
10. 隋書
11. 全元起

77

Wang Ping lived at the period of Pao Ying.[12] However, he stated that he had obtained a well-preserved ancient edition by means of which he was able to supplement the missing roll. According to the commentary written by Lin I[13] and others in the Sung dynasty, it is stated that those rolls following the "Treatise on the Plan of the Heavenly Measurements"[14] were voluminous, and quite different from the other fascicles of the Su Wên, and (the commentators) suspected that those represented the great *Treatise of Yin and Yang* which was mentioned in the preface of Chang Chi's *Treatise on Typhoid Fever* and which was used by Wang Ping to supplement the lost roll. This assumption is, perhaps, reasonable. (The fascicles) on "The Methods of Acupuncture"[15] and "Innate Diseases"[16] were lost and could not be supplied again even in the edition of (Wang) Ping.

The order of the fascicles was changed considerably in the edition of Wang Ping. But underneath the title of each fascicle it is stated what position this chapter had originally occupied in the edition of Ch'üan Yüan-ch'i. Thus we can still find the old arrangement

The commentaries of Wang Ping reached the most profound points and were full of discoveries. Wang Ping said: "The great cold one feels in times of great heat is cold—one has no water. The great heat one feels in times of great cold is heat—one has no fire. He who has no fire should not remove his water but should increase the sources of his natural fire in order to disperse the shade of Yin. He who has no water should not reduce his fire but should increase the force of his water in order to control the light of Yang." This led to the school of profound investigation of the gates of life[17] of Hsüeh Chi[18] and others in the Ming dynasty, and expresses a deep knowledge of the principles of medicine.

The name of (Wang) Ping was recorded in the genealogical table of prime ministers in the *New History of the T'ang Dynasty*, and his official title was recorded as "military councillor to the mayor of the

---

12. 762 A.D., T'ang dynasty.
13. Lin I 林億 also superintended the revised publication of the *Meh Ching* or "Classic of the Pulse" in 1068.
14. 天元紀大論
15. 刺法論
16. 本病論
17. 探本命門
18. 薛己

capital." But Lin I said that, according to the *Jên Wu Chih*,[19] Wang Ping was one of the highest ministers (of the T'ang dynasty).[20] We do not know which is right. All students of medicine, however, call Wang Ping "Minister Wang"[21] because they are familiar with the book of Lin I.

The (ideographs for) the name of Wang Ping were recorded as 王 砅 in the *Record of Books*[22] of Chao Kung-wu.[23] In the works of Tu Fu[24] there was a poem which was sent to his distant cousin Wang Ping (王 砅) and (the writing of) this name was identical with the name mentioned in the *Record of Books*. But in all other works of the T'ang and Sung dynasties the (commentator's) name was written as 冰, and even in an edition (of the *Nei Ching*) which was published in the Sung dynasty the name was written as 冰. It is probable that Chao Kung-wu was mistaken when he followed the poem of Tu Fu.[25]

19. The *Jên Wu Chih* (人 物 志) was composed by Liu Shao during the third century A.D. It is divided into twelve sections and it treats of the divisions of mankind into classes. (Wylie, *Notes on Chinese Literature*, p. 158.)
20. 太 僕 令
21. 王 太 僕
22. 讀 書 志
23. 晁 公 武 twelfth century A.D. From 1165 he was prefect at Hsing-yüan in Shensi. (Giles, *Biographical Dictionary*, p. 85 *s.v.* Chao Kung-wu.)
24. 杜 甫 A.D. 712–770. One of China's most famous poets.
25. The argument in this paragraph refers only to the written form of the annotator's name "Ping." Both forms 砅 and 冰 are pronounced alike.

APPENDIX II

An Introduction to the *Yellow Emperor's Canon of Internal Medicine*

Composed by the
Master Who Opens Up Mysteries, Wang Ping (啓 玄 子 王 冰)

VERILY, the releasing of bondages, the overcoming of troubles, the preservation of one's natural state, the proper direction of the breath, the raising of the great multitude to benevolence and long life, the guiding of the feeble and weak to attain tranquillity can be accomplished only by the methods of the three [first] sages [mentioned below]. The K'ung An-kuo preface to the *Book of History* says that the writings of Fu-hsi,[1] Shên-nung,[2] and Huang-ti were called the "Three Mounds."[3] They discussed the great Way. Pan Ku[4] in the "Treatise on the Canons and Literature" of his *History of the Former Han Dynasty* [Han Shu][5] lists the *Yellow Emperor's Canon of Internal Medicine* in 18 rolls. "Simple Questions" (Su-wên) represented 9 rolls of that *Canon*; together with the 9 rolls in the "Mystical Pivot" (*Ling Shu*) they made up the [exact] number [of the rolls in that book].

Although the years have changed and the age is different, these [words] have been held together and have been taught as subject of study, so that [this book] is still preserved. It was feared that the wrong person [might secure this information], hence at times this book was hidden. And thus the seventh roll was hidden by Mr. Shih and the book which we respectfully take now has only 8 rolls.

1. Fu-hsi, who is said to have lived about 2800 B.C., is the first of the five rulers of the legendary period of China's history. To him is attributed the invention of the Eight Diagrams (*Pa Kua* 八 卦). These diagrams are a pictorial representation of the Chinese universalistic philosophy. Their broken and unbroken lines are interpreted to explain the working of all natural phenomena.
2. Shên-nung is the second of the legendary emperors. He is said to have lived about 2700 B.C. He is called the Divine Husbandman and is venerated as the father of agriculture. In that capacity he is reputed to have tasted all herbs in order to acquaint himself with their value. To him is commonly attributed the writing of the *Herbal* (Pên Tsao 本 草).
3. This phrase can be found in the *Tso Chuan*. See Legge, *Chinese Classics*, p. 641b.
4. A.D. 32–92.
5. 30: 78b in Wang Sien-chien's edition.

Be that as it may, yet its style is concise, its ideas are vast, its principles are deep, and its goal is profound. The phenomena of heaven and earth are distinguished, the state of Yin and Yang is set forth, the causes for change and metamorphosis are exhibited, and the symptoms of death or continued life are made plain. It is not necessary to ponder [upon these principles], they are in harmony far and near, the implicit and the explicit are in perfect accord. If you examine the words in this document, you will find that they contain proof; if you test its facts there will be no errors, so that it can really be called the source of the first principle and the beginning of [the process of] preserving one's life. Even if one should have spontaneous natural talents, deep and profound and wonderful knowledge, nevertheless we are still in need of textual and philological elucidations to put (our knowledge) into exemplary form. One does not walk if there is no path and one does not leave if there is no door.

Yet if one concentrates one's attention upon the research on the essence and traces the implicit and hidden sources of things, or knows the truly important features of this document, then (if he sees) that the eyes of an ox are without perfection, he will be successful as if he had the "mysterious assistance of the spirits and gods."[6] Moreover people who are famous for a generation and remarkable heroes appear from time to time. Thus in the Chou dynasty there was his excellency Ch'in,[7] in the Han dynasty there was his excellency Ch'un-yü,[8] in the Wei dynasty there was his excellency Chang[9] and his excellency Hua[10]—all of these were persons who attained this marvelous way. All of them daily renewed their usefulness and greatly aided the multitude of people, their famous deeds benefitting mankind just as brilliant foliage lends glory to blossoms, their reputation matched their action. In all probability the fame of the teaching was also the bestowal of Heaven.

6. A phrase from the *Book of Changes*, App. V.1; tr. by Legge, *Chinese Classics*, p. 444.
7. Ch'in Yüeh-jên 秦 越 人 about 225 B.C. commonly held to be identical with the famous physician Pien Ch'iao 扁 鵲 whose dates are uncertain; anecdotes about him extend from the fifth century B.C. to the second century B.C.
8. Ch'un-yü I 淳 于 意 born B.C. 205, distinguished for his knowledge of medicine. In B.C. 180 he was appointed to be court physician.
9. Chang (Tao)-ling 張 道 陵 A.D 34–156. The founder of religious Taoism.
10. Hua T'o 華 陀, a famous physician and surgeon; died A.D. 220; cf. *Hou-Han-shu* Em. 72B: 5b–9a.

I, [Wang] Ping, in my youth admired the Way and always loved the care of one's health. Fortunately I happened to come upon the true Canon [of the Yellow Emperor], whose function was that of a mirror which foretells the future. But the popular copies were disordered, there were duplications in the tables of contents, the first and the last [parts of the book] contradicted [each other], the words and their meaning were disparate, so that it was difficult to apply [its teaching] and to read and understand it was also difficult. These [errors] have been retained for years and months and they have been repeated so that they have produced corruptions [of the text]. Sometimes one fascicle appeared twice and at the other place it was given a different title. Sometimes two discussions were combined and to both was given one heading. Sometimes when the answer to a question had not yet been completed, there was set up the title of a separate fascicle. Sometimes the slips for writing had disappeared or were not written out, and it said [for example], "This age lacks [such and such materials]." The chapter of "the Canon"[11] was twice combined [with other material] and was put ahead of [the chapter on] "the needle"[12] and "the stomach"[13] and its reading was uncertain. "The proper recipe"[14] was absorbed and became the fascicle on "the cough."[15] "Unreality and reality"[16] was separated and was made into "going contrary to and according to."[17] [Material] was added to "the preparation of the warp"[18] and it was made into a "discussion"; "the important features,"[19] "the moderation"[20] and "the skin section"[21] became "blood-vessels";[22] thus the loftiest teaching was held back and the use of the needle[23] was put in front. Matters of this sort were countless.

Anyone who desires to ascend the T'ai Yo[24] cannot succeed without a road; anyone who wishes to travel to Fu Sang[25] cannot arrive

11. Fascicle 62. 17. Fascicle 64.
12. Fascicle 54. 18. Fascicle 57.
13. Fascicle 40. 19. Fascicle 50.
14. Fascicle 12. 20. Fascicle 55.
15. Fascicle 38. 21. Fascicle 56.
16. Fascicle 28. 22. Fascicle 57.
23. Acupuncture.
24. T'ai Yo 岱嶽, an ancient name of T'ai Shan, the chief of the five sacred mountains of China situated in Shantung.
25. Fu Sang 扶桑, a mythical country eastward of China. The emperor Shih Huang-ti fitted out an expedition of young men and maidens to seek this land in 219 B.C. Gradually, as for instance in the records of the Sui dynasty, Fu Sang was identified with Japan.

there without a ship.   There have been men who have made diligent and intensive investigations [of original texts].   After twelve years of study I now understand the principles; I inquired into the right points and into the wrong points and [the results] satisfy my old desire.

I received the original [secret, hidden] edition of the foremost master, his excellency Chang[26] at the home of my teacher Kuo Tzu Chai.[27]   The writing in this text is very clear, the principles and the reasoning in his text are well-rounded; and by making use of it for purposes of interpretation many doubtful points have disappeared like ice.   As I am afraid that his text may be lost in my hands and that, as a consequence, the teaching material will disappear, I wrote a commentary to it in order to perpetuate it eternally.   I combined it with the texts in my possession into one book of eighty-one fascicles (篇) and twenty-four rolls (卷).   It is my intention to investigate the tail in order to understand the head, to investigate the commentaries in order to understand the classic, to develop the (medical knowledge) for the young men, and to spread widely the highest principles.

Some paragraphs of this book [original text] are missing and its writing is interrupted, hence the meaning of the different paragraphs cannot be combined.   I tried to find the missing parts from other classics and essays and transplanted them in order to fill the gaps. In this [original] edition some titles and topics have been lost, and there is no clarity in the explanations, thus I guessed their meanings and clarified them by adding words.   There is also some confusion in regard to different parts of fascicles and their contents; in such cases of confusion the contents of the successive sentences are not related to each other, and sometimes there are titles missing; hence I divided and arranged them according to classifications and gave them new titles.

The text consists of conversation of the emperor with his minister. These conversations are not always in accordance with etiquette; in such cases I added some words in order to shed light upon their exalted and humble position.   There are also some wrong paragraphs and confused characters and those which are overlapping; I attempted to determine their meaning and omitted those confused

26. Chang Chung-ching.   See Appendix I, footnote 4.
27. 享 子 齋

and overlapping parts in order to preserve the essential portions. The meaning of some words is very deeply hidden and it is difficult to explain them roughly, hence I am writing another book by the name of *Pearls of Mystery* to explain the meanings.[28]   All the words which were added by me are written in red, the purpose of which is to distinguish between the new and the old and to prevent confusion between the words.

[All my efforts are made with the purpose of] clarifying [the text to fulfil] the loyal hopes and wishes [of the Emperor] and to bring out the profound words [or the original text] in such a way that they are like stars suspended high [in Heaven] where K'uei cannot be confused with Chang,[29] and [in such a way] that they are like a deep well which is so clear that one can distinguish scales and shells. [I also wish] to prevent the Emperor and his subordinates from dying young; and to give to both, the barbarians and the Chinese, the hope of prolonging their lives; and to clarify matters for the students; and to make the highest Tao prevail; and to keep in continuous existence the highest principles, so that after a thousand years the people shall know that the wisdom and kindness of the great sages were without limits.

This preface was written in the first year of Pao Ying[30] of the great T'ang dynasty.

This [edition of Wang Ping] was corrected by Sun Chao (孫 兆).

This edition was also read by Kao Pao-hêng (高 保 衡), Sun Ch'i (孫 奇), and Lin I (林 億).[31]

---

28. According to the "Newly Revised Edition," the *Pearls of Mystery* (Hsüan Chu 玄 珠) has disappeared.   There are ten rolls (卷) of the *Hsüan Chu* and three rolls of the *Chao Ming Yin Chih* existing, but these books were written by some author later than Wang Ping.   Although these books are not the work of Wang Ping, they nevertheless furnish explanations to volumes nineteen to twenty-two of the *Su Wên*.   The three volumes of the *Chao Ming Yin Chih* (昭 明 隱 旨) and the *T'ien Yüan Yü Ts'e* (天 元 玉 冊) complement each other but differ in many places from the principles expounded by Wang Ping.

29. Two of the twenty-eight zodiacal signs.

30. 762 A.D.

31. Eleventh century A.D.

APPENDIX III

Introduction to the Enlarged Complementary Edition of the *Huang Ti Nei Ching Su Wên*

I [your humble servant] hear that not to forget dangers at times of security and not to forget decline or fall at times of safe existence constituted the most important duties of the early sages. (I hear) that to search for the ailments of the people and to sympathize with the distress of the people represented the profound humaneness of the superior rulers.

In ancient times when Huang Ti ascended the throne, he ruled his empire by the principle that the body is connected with the rest. Sitting in the Bright Hall,[1] looking down upon the eight poles, and investigating the five constant (virtues), he thought: When man is born he carries the Yin and embraces the Yang; [he thought] that [man] ate [food of different] flavors and wore [clothes of different] colors; [he thought] that from the outside man was disturbed by cold and heat, that internally man was continually moved by happiness and anger, and that throughout the history of our country there had been many who had died young.

To gather in time the five blessings and to distribute them widely to all the people, Huang Ti, accompanied by Ch'i Po, investigated upwards into the rules of Heaven, and downwards they thoroughly investigated the principles of the Earth; from distant places they selected [rules and regulations] concerning beings; in near places they selected [rules and regulations] concerning their own bodies; they questioned each other, then they established rules [of medical knowledge] which were to bring happiness to ten thousand generations.

Then men like Lei Kung[2] could receive knowledge and pass it on,

---

1. 明 堂 The complete meaning of this term is unclear to Chinese as well as western sinologues. See J. J. M. de Groot, *The Religious System of China*, its ancient forms, evolution, history and present aspect, manners, customs and social institutions connected therewith (6 vols., Leyden, 1892–1910), III, 1362.
2. 雷 公 , one of the disciples of Huang-ti. Seven chapters of the *Nei Ching* are attributed to him. See Wong and Wu, *History of Chinese Medicine*, p. 6. Dr. Alfred Forke in his

and thus the *Canon of Internal Medicine* was written. It was treasured by every dynasty [generation] and was never lost. At the time of the Chou dynasty there was a man whose name was (Ch'in) Ho (秦 和); he handed down the theory of the six breaths which was recorded clearly in the *Tso Chuan*.³ Later one or two tenths [of the *Nei Ching*] were received by Yüeh-jên⁴ and he developed them in the *Nan Ching*.⁵ At the time of the former Han dynasty, Chung-ching⁶ wrote a book⁷ which concerned itself with the missing doctrines implied in the *Nei Ching*. At the time of the Chin dynasty, Huang-fu Mi⁸ arranged [the knowledge he had received from the *Nei Ching*] into the *Chia I*.⁹ At the time of the Sui dynasty Yang Shang-shan made use of this knowledge by editing the *T'ai Su*.¹⁰ At the same time there was Ch'üan Yüan-ch'i,¹¹ who began the work of writing a commentary to the *Nei Ching*, but the seventh roll was lost.

In the time of Pao Yin [762 A.D.], in the T'ang dynasty, one of the highest ministers,¹² Wang Ping, became very interested in this work. He received the volumes which had been preserved by a former master [of medicine, Chang Chung-ching¹³] and he edited and commentated them to a large extent. These (volumes which he had received) still constituted the original text of the three emperors¹⁴ and were brilliant reading. Unfortunately, it was decreed that this work should be classified as a medical book and should be given over to the craftsmen; gentlemen [men of higher education]

Geschichte der Alten Chinesischen Philosophie (Hamburg, 1927), p. 244, identifies Lei Kung with Ch'i Po, Huang-ti's minister and collaborator on the *Nei Ching*.

3. 左 傳 , Tso Ch'iu-ming's (or Tso-ch'iu Ming) important commentary on the *Ch'un Ch'iu* 春 秋 "Springs and Autumns," the title of the last literary work of Confucius.

4. See Appendix II, footnote 7.

5. 難 經 , the so-called "Difficult Classic," a treatise which is attributed to Pien Ch'iao who wrote it with the purpose of elucidating the *Huang Ti Nei Ching Su Wên*.

6. See Appendix I, footnote 4.

7. The *Treatise on Typhoid Fever*.

8. See Appendix I, footnote 6.

9. *Ibid.*

10. 太 素 "The Beginning of Substance" (Taoist).

11. 全 元 起

12. See Appendix I, footenote 20.

13. See Appendix II, footnote 26, and Appendix I, footnote 4.

14. This refers to the three of the five legendary emperors who are venerated as the highest gods of medicine. See Appendix II, footnotes 1 and 2.

would seldom refer to it.[15]   The distance [in time] from the sages is great and the methods [contained in this book] have become unclear; thus text and commentaries have become disarranged and its principles have become confused.

[Those men of the T'ang dynasty who classified this work as a medical book] really did not know that the principles of the three classics of the three emperors of the ancient times—the lofty deeds of emperors and kings, the able conduct of the sages and the men of virtue, [the principles] of the Emperor Yao[16] of the T'ang dynasty who arranged the four seasons, [the principles of] the Emperor Shun[17] of the Yü dynasty who regularized the seven heavenly bodies, [the principles of] the Great Yü[18] who regulated the six ministries of government[19] in order to revive the emperor's position, the [principles of] Wên Wang[20] who assigned his six sons to the task of clarification of the trigrams,[21] [the principles of] I Yin[22] who blended the five flavors to gain the recognition of the Emperor, and [the principles of] Chi Tzu[23] who arranged the five elements to be helpful to the world— [they did not know] that all these principles were alike.   How could they give the most essential and the most delicate methods to the lowest and most humble of men?   Oh, it was truly fortunate that the book was not lost!

In the time of Chia Yu[24] the Emperor Jên Tsung feared that the heritage of the holy emperors should fall to the ground, hence his Majesty decreed that the scholars who had medical knowledge should correct the text [of the *Nei Ching*].   We, the servants, were

15. Physicians were considered craftsmen and held a low social position.

16. 堯 }
17. 舜 } Three ancient rulers during the "golden age" of Chinese history.
18. 禹 }

19. 六府

20. 文 王 B.C. 1182–1135, known as the Duke of Chou, the father of the first sovereign of the Chou dynasty.

21. Pa Kua (八 卦) Although the invention of the eight trigrams is commonly attributed to the Emperor Fu Hsi, it is more likely that they were conceived by Wên Wang, the author of the *I Ching*, "The Book of Changes," in which are recorded the theories of the trigrams which are held to disclose the solution for every problem in life.

22. 伊 尹 eighteenth century B.C. He was a minister under the first emperor of the Shang dynasty. Giles, *Biographical Dictionary*, *s.v.* I Yin.

23. 箕 子 twelfth century B.C., one of the foremost nobles under the last emperor of the Yin dynasty. To him is attributed the authorship of the "Great Plan," a part of the *Canon of History*. Giles, *Biographical Dictionary*, *s.v.* Chi Tzu.

24. 嘉 祐 1056 A.D.; Sung dynasty.

charged with the duty of administration and correction. After ten years of study we have investigated [the text] as to its internal [contents] and to its external [meaning]; we have collected many different editions; we have tried to understand their meaning and we have corrected errors [of the *Nei Ching*]; thirty or forty per cent [of these errors] were corrected, but the rest could not be mastered. We thought that this was not sufficient to reward the wise order and to answer the sacred wishes [of the Emperor]; therefore we once more took up the books of the Han and T'ang dynasties which dealt with ancient medical knowledge and which still exist in the present day; and we obtained several tens of them of which we made an account on the basis of which we corrected our text. After thorough investigation we connected many points, we made many deductions [which brought about] a full understanding. Sometimes we began from the root in order to explore the branches; sometimes we began from the tributary in order to find out the origin of the river; thus we found out what could be found out, and arranged it according to the topics. More than six thousand words have now been corrected and more than two thousand comments. The adoption or omission of each word must have its foundation. All those mistaken paragraphs and unclear meanings have thus been clarified.

If we use the [contents] of this book to rule our body we can prevent disasters before they begin; if we apply this book to statesmanship we can enlarge and prolong life without limits. We sincerely thank His Majesty the Emperor who rules over the destiny of the entire world, who holds a position without bounds, who is a successor to the wishes of the former emperors and who fulfilled [these wishes], who revived the neglected study and corrected it in the right way, so that there will be harmony, that there will not arise any disasters and that all the people in the world will approach a long life.

Respectfully submitted by Kao Pao-hêng (高 保 衡), Physician of the Imperial University, and Lin I (林 億), Minister in Charge of the Privy Council   [1056–1066, Sung Dynasty].

BIBLIOGRAPHY

Books and reference works in Chinese

Chung-kuo jên-ming ta-tz'u-tien (中 國 人 名 大 辭 典) [Biographical encyclopedia of Chinese names]. Shanghai, 1923.

Chung-kuo ti-ming ta-tz'u-tien (中 國 地 名 大 辭 典) [Chinese geographical dictionary]. Peking, 1930.

K'ang-hsi tzu-tien (康 熙 字 典), compiled under K'ang-hsi (1662–1723). Shanghai, [1904].

Kuo-wên ch'êng-yü tz'u-tien (國 文 成 語 辭 典) [Dictionary of quotations and proverbs in literary Chinese]. Shanghai, 1926.

Shu-mu ta-wên (書 目 答 問) [Bibliography of important Chinese books], compiled by Chang Chih-tung (1837–1909). Shanghai, 1925.

Shuo-wên chieh-tzu (說 文 解 字) [The analysis of ideographs], compiled about A.D. 100. Shanghai, n.d.

Ssu-k'u ch'üan-shu tsung-mu t'i-yao (四 庫 全 書 總 目 提 要) [A complete bibliography of the most important works], compiled under the auspices of the Chinese government in 1772. Shanghai, 1933.

Sung-yüan i-lai su-tzu-p'u (宋 元 以 來 俗 字 譜) [Compendium of popular forms of characters in use since the Sung and Yüan dynasties]. Shanghai, 1930.

Tzu-shih Ching-hua (子 史 精 華) [Lexicon of quotations and proverbs from the works of famous philosophers and historians]. Shanghai, [1922].

Tz'u-yüan (辭 源) [Chinese encyclopedic dictionary]. Shanghai, 1916.

Books and Articles Dealing with
The History of Chinese Medicine

Bretschneider, Emilii Vasil'evich. *Botanicum Sinicum*, Notes on Chinese botany from native and Western sources. London, 1882.

Cleyer, Andreas. *Specimen medicinae Sinicae*. Frankfurt, 1662.

Cohn, W., "Anatomie in China," *Deutsche Medizinische Wochenschrift*, 1899, No. 30.

Cowdry, E. V., "A Comparison of Ancient Chinese Anatomical Charts with the 'Fünfbilderserie' of Sudhoff," *Anatomical Record*, XXII (1921), 1–25.

——, "Taoist Ideas of Anatomy," *Annals of Medical History*, III (1921), 301–309.

Dabry, P. *La Médecine chez les Chinois*, ouvrage corrigé et précédé d'une préface par M. J. Léon Soubeiran. Paris, 1863.

Dawson, Percy M., "Su-wên, the Basis of Chinese Medicine," *Annals of Medical History*, VII (1925), 59–64.

Eckstein, Oskar, "Über Altchinesische Medizin," *Schweizerische Medizinische Wochenschrift*, 1925, No. 15, pp. 1–8. (reprint vol. 8, Hauer Collection)

Fujikawa, Y. *Japanese Medicine*, tr. from the German by John Ruhräh. New York, 1934. (Clio Medica)

Gruenhagen, "Die Grundlagen der Chinesischen Medizin," *Janus, Archives Internationales pour l'Histoire de la Médecine et la Géographie Médicale*, XIII (1908) 1–14, 121–137, 191–205, 268–278, 328–337.

Du Halde, J. P., "The Art of Medicine among the Chinese," in *A Description of the Empire of China* (4 vols., London, 1736), II..

Hsieh, E. T., "A Review of Ancient Chinese Anatomy," *Anatomical Record*, XX (1921), No. 1, 97–127.

Hübotter, Franz. *Die Chinesische Medizin zu Beginn des XX. Jahrhunderts und ihr Historischer Entwicklungsgang.* Leipzig, 1929. (China Bibliothek der "Asia Major," Bd. I)

——, "Zwei Berühmte Chinesische Ärzte des Altertums," *Mitteilungen der Deutschen Gesellschaft für Natur- und Völkerkunde Ostasiens*, XXI (Tokyo, 1925), Teil A.

Huizenga, Lee S., "Lü Tsu and his Relation to Other Medicine Gods," *Chinese Medical Journal*, LVIII (1940), 275–283.

Hume, Edward H. *The Chinese Way in Medicine.* Baltimore, 1940.

——, *Doctors East, Doctors West.* New York, 1946.

——, "Some Foundations of Chinese Medicine," *Chinese Medical Journal*, LXI (1942), 291–298.

Latourette, K. S. *A Century of Protestant Missions in China.* Shanghai, 1907.

Lee Tao, "Ten Celebrated Physicians and their Temple," *Chinese Medical Journal*, LVIII (1940), 267–274.

Li, Shih-chên. *Chinese Materia Medica*, tr. by Bernard E. Read, from the *Pen ts'ao kang mu*, A.D. 1597. Peiping, 1931–32.

Lockhart, W. *The Medical Missionary in China.* 8 vols., London, 1861.

Macgowan, D. J. *History of Medicine in China.* Chinese Imper. Cust. Med. Report. Shanghai, 1882.

Maspero, Henri, "Les Procédés de 'Nourir le Principe Vital' dans la Religion Taoiste Ancienne," *Journal Asiatique*, CCXXIX (1937), 177–252, 353–430.

"The Medical Missionary Society in China," Address with Minutes and Proceedings. Canton, 1838.

Morse, William R. *Chinese Medicine.* New York, 1934. (Clio Medica)

Nakayama, T. *Acupuncture et Médecine Chinoise Vérifiées au Japon*, traduites du japonais par T. Sakurazawa et G. Soulié de Morant et précédées d'une préface de G. Soulié de Morant. Paris, 1934.

Okada, W., "Das Japanische Medicinalwesen und die Socialen Verhältnisse der Japanischen Ärzte," *Vierteljahrsschrift f. gerichtl. Medizin und Öfentl. Sanitätswesen*, XVIII (3rd ser.), H. 1.

Read, Bernard E., "Gleanings from Old Chinese Medicine," *Annals of Medical History*, VIII (1926), 16–19.

Smith, Frederick Porter. *Chinese Materia Medica; Vegetable Kingdom*, extensively rev. from Dr. F. Porter Smith's work by Rev. G. A. Stuart, M.D. Shanghai, 1911.

Soulié de Morant, G. *Précis de la Vraie Acuponcture Chinoise.* Paris, 1935.

Töply, Robert (Ritter von), "Die Medizin in China," *Balneologische Zentralzeitung*, 1902, Nos. 43–45.

Wang Chi-min, "China's Contribution to Medicine in the Past," *Annals of Medical History*, VIII (1926), 192–201.

Whitney, W. Norton, "Notes on the History of Medical Progress in Japan," *Transactions of the Asiatic Society of Japan*, (Yokohama, 1885), 245–269.

Wong, K. C., and Lien-teh Wu. *History of Chinese Medicine*. Tientsin, [1932?].

Woost, Georg Edward. *Quaedam de acupunctura Orientalium ex oblivionis tenebris ab Europaeis medicis nuper revocata*. Lipsiae, [1826].

Wu, Lien-teh, "Past and Present Trends in the Medical History of China," *Chinese Medical Journal*, LIII (1938), 313–322.

Dictionaries and Reference Books and Works on Chinese Philosophy, Religion, and History

Albright, William Foxwell. *From the Stone Age to Christianity*. Baltimore, 1940.

Chalmers, John. *An Account of the Structures of Chinese Characters under 300 Primary Forms after the Shwoh-wan, 100, A.D., and the Phonetic Shwoh-wan, 1833*. Shanghai, 1911.

Cordier, Henri. *Bibliotheca Sinica. Dictionnaire Bibliographique des Ouvrages Relatifs à l'Empire Chinois*. 2 vols., Paris, 1904–1908.

Couling, Samuel. *The Encyclopedia Sinica*. London, 1917.

Couvreur, F. Séraphin. *Dictionnaire Classique de la Langue Chinoise*. Ho Kien Fu, 1911.

Doré, Henri. *Manuel des Superstitions Chinoises*, un petit indicateur des superstitions, les plus communes en Chine. Shanghai, 1926.

Dvorak, Rudolf. *Chinas Religionen. Zweiter Teil: Lao-tsi und seine Lehre*. Münster i.W., 1903. (Darstellungen aus dem Gebiete der nichtchristlichen Religionsgeschichte, XV)

Fitzgerald, C. P. *China, A Short Cultural History*. New York, 1938.

Forke, Alfred. *Geschichte der Alten Chinesischen Philosophie*. Hamburg, 1927. (Hamburgische Universität, Abhandlungen aus dem Gebiet der Auslandskunde, Bd. 25)

———. *The World Conception of the Chinese: their Astronomical, Cosmological and Physico-Philosophical Speculations*. London, 1925.

Franke, Otto, "Die Chinesen," in Chantepie de la Saussure, *Religionsgeschichte* (Tübingen, 1925), Aufl. 4, Bd. I, pp. 193–261.

Giles, Herbert Allen. *A Biographical Dictionary*. London, 1898.

———. *A Chinese English Dictionary*. 2nd ed., London, 1912.

———. *A Glossary of Reference on Subjects Connected with the Far East*. 3rd ed., Shanghai, 1900.

Granet, Marcel. *La Religion des Chinois*. Paris, 1922.

Groot, J. J. M. de. *Chinesische Urkunden zur Geschichte Asiens*, in vollstaendiger Zusammenfassung übersetzt und erläutert. 2 vols., Berlin and Leipzig, 1921–1926.

———. *Universismus, die Grundlage der Religion und Ethik, des Staatswesens und der Wissenschaften Chinas*. Berlin, 1918.

Grube, Wilhelm. "Religion der Alten Chinesen," in A. Bertholet, *Religionsgeschichtliches Lesebuch* (5 vols., Tübingen, 1908).

Grube, Wilhelm. *Religion und. Kultus der Chinesen.* Leipzig, 1910.

Hackmann, Heinrich. *Chinesische Philosophie.* München, 1927.

Hersey, John, "Hiroshima," *The New Yorker*, August 31, 1946.

——, "The Red Pepper Village," *Life*, August 26, 1946, pp. 92–100, 102, 105.

Krause, F. E. A. *Ju-Tao-Fo . . . die Religiösen und Philosophischen Systeme Ostasiens.* München, 1924.

Legge, James. *The Chinese Classics*, with translation, critical notes, prolegomena and copious indexes. 7 vols., Oxford, 1893–1895.

Littré, Emile. *Dictionnaire de la Langue Francaise.* Paris, 1881.

Maspero, Henri. *La Chine Antique.* Paris, 1927.

Mathews, R. H. *A Chinese-English Dictionary*, revised American edition. Cambridge, Mass., 1944.

Morse, H. B. *The Chronicles of the East India Company Trading to China, 1635–1843.* Oxford, 1929.

Pan Ku. *The History of the Former Han Dynasty*, a critical translation with annotations by Homer H. Dubs, with the collaboration of Jen T'ai and P'an Lo-chi. Baltimore, 1938.

Rémusat, Jean Pierre Abel, "De la Philosophie Chinoise," in *Mélanges Posthumes d'Histoire et de Littérature Orientales* (Paris, 1843), pp. 160–205.

Rudd, Herbert F. *Chinese Social Origins.* Chicago, 1928.

Saussure, Léopold de. *Les Origines de l'Astronomie Chinoise.* London, [n.d.].

Ssu-ma Ch'ien. *Les Mémoires Historiques de Se-ma-Ts'ien*, traduits et annotés par Edouard Chavannes. 5 vols., Paris, 1895–1905.

Suzuki, Daisetz Teitaro. *A Brief History of Early Chinese Philosophy.* London, 1914. (Probsthain's Oriental Series, VII)

Van Aalst, J. A. *Chinese Music.* Shanghai and London, 1884.

Werner, G. T. C. *A History of Chinese Civilization. The Shanghai Times*, 1940. Vol. 1.

Wieger, Léon. *Histoire des Croyances Religieuses et des Opinions Philosophiques depuis l'Origine jusqu'à nos Jours.* Ho Kien Fu, 1922.

——. *Leçons Etymologiques.* Sienhsien, [1923?].

——. *Chinese Characters, their Origin, Etymology, History, Classification and Signification*, a thorough study from Chinese documents, tr. into English by L. Davrout. Ho Kien Fu, Catholic Mission Press, 1915; Peking, 1940.

——. *Rudiments* [de parler et de style chinois]. [Ho Kien Fu], n.d.

Wilhelm II, German Emperor. *Die Chinesische Monade, Ihre Geschichte und Ihre Deutung.* Leipzig, 1934.

Wilhelm, Richard. *Geschichte der Chinesischen Kultur.* München, [1928].

——. *Lao-tse und der Taoismus.* Stuttgart, 1925.

Williams, Ch. A. Speed. *Outlines of Chinese Symbolism.* Peiping, 1931.

Wylie, A. *Notes on Chinese Literature.* Shanghai, 1922.

Zenker, Ernst Victor. *Geschichte der Chinesischen Philosophie*, das klassische Zeitalter bis zur Han Dynastie (206 v. Chr.). Reichenberg, 1926.

Translation

of the

Huang Ti Nei Ching Su Wên

[The Yellow Emperor's Classic on Internal Medicine]

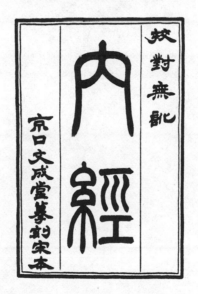

Title-Page of the
Huang Ti Nei Ching Su Wên

Book 1

1. *Treatise on the Natural Truth in Ancient Times*

In ancient times when the Yellow Emperor was born he was endowed with divine talents; while yet in early infancy he could speak; while still very young he was quick of apprehension and penetrating; when he was grown up he was sincere and comprehending; when he became perfect he ascended to Heaven.[1]

The Yellow Emperor once addressed T'ien Shih,[2] the divinely inspired teacher: "I have heard that in ancient times the people lived (through the years) to be over a hundred years, and yet they remained active and did not become decrepit in their activities. But nowadays people reach only half of that age and yet become decrepit and failing. Is it because the world changes from generation to generation? Or is it that mankind is becoming negligent (of the laws of nature)?"

Ch'i Po answered: "In ancient times those people who understood Tao [the way of self cultivation] patterned themselves upon the Yin and the Yang [the two principles in nature] and they lived in harmony with the arts of divination.[3]

"There was temperance in eating and drinking. Their hours of rising and retiring were regular and not disorderly and wild. By these means the ancients kept their bodies united with their souls, so as to fulfill their allotted span completely, measuring unto a hundred years before they passed away.

"Nowadays people are not like this; they use wine as beverage and they adopt recklessness as usual behaviour. They enter the cham-

1. See also: Edouard Chavannes, *Les Mémoires historiques de Sema Ts'ien* (Paris, 1885), p. 26.
2. 天 師 This title when applied to formal Taoism means "Master of Heaven" and denotes the highest rank in the Taoist hierarchy. See W. Grube, *Religion and Kultus der Chinesen* (Leipzig, 1910), p. 115.
3. Fung Yu-lan, *A History of Chinese Philosophy*, tr. by Derk Bodde (Peipin, 1937), p. 26. Wang Ping says: 術 數 are the great rules of the protection of life. These characters, translated by J. J. M. de Groot as "Kunstrechnen" (*Universismus*, p. 321), are the name of an ancient science combining astrology and divination. The chronomancy of the calendar represents one of the phases of these artful calculations.

ber (of love) in an intoxicated condition;[4] their passions exhaust their
vital forces; their cravings dissipate their true (essence); they do
not know how to find contentment within themselves; they are not
skilled in the control of their spirits. They devote all their attention
to the amusement of their minds, thus cutting themselves off from
the joys of long (life). Their rising and retiring is without regularity.
For these reasons they reach only one half of the hundred years
and then they degenerate.

"In the most ancient times the teachings of the sages (聖 人) were
followed by those beneath them; they said that weakness and noxious
influences and injurious winds should be avoided at specific times.
They [the sages] were tranquilly content in nothingness and the true
vital force accompanied them always; their vital (original) spirit was
preserved within, thus, how could illness come to them!

"They exercised restraint of their wills and reduced their desires;
their hearts were at peace and without any fear; their bodies toiled
and yet did not become weary.

"Their spirit followed in harmony and obedience; everything was
satisfactory to their wishes and they could achieve whatever they
wished. Any kind of food was beautiful (to them);[5] and any kind
of clothing was satisfactory. They felt happy under any condition.
To them it did not matter whether a man held a high or a low position
in life. These men can be called pure at heart. No kind of desire
can tempt the eyes of those pure people and their mind cannot be
misled by excessiveness and evil.

"(In such a society) no matter whether men are wise or foolish,
virtuous or bad, they are without fear of anything; they are in
harmony with Tao, the Right Way. Thus they could live more
than one hundred years and remain active without becoming decrepit, because their virtue was perfect and never imperiled."

The Emperor asked: "When people grow old then they cannot
give birth to children. Is it because they have exhausted their
strength in depravity or is it because of natural fate?"

Ch'i Po answered: "When a girl is seven years of age, the emanations of the kidneys (腎 氣) become abundant, she begins to change
her teeth and her hair grows longer. When she reaches her four-
teenth year she begins to menstruate and is able to become pregnant

4. Wang Ping says: They overindulge.
5. Wang Ping explains: They were satisfied with good food as well as bad food.

and the movement in the great thoroughfare pulse (太 衝 脉) is strong.[6] Menstruation comes at regular times, thus the girl is able to give birth to a child.

"When the girl reaches the age of twenty-one years the emanations of the kidneys are regular, the last tooth has come out, and she is fully grown. When the woman reaches the age of twenty-eight, her muscles and bones are strong, her hair has reached its full length and her body is flourishing and fertile.

"When the woman reaches the age of thirty-five, the pulse indicating [the region of] the 'Sunlight' (陽 明) deteriorates, her face begins to wrinkle and her hair begins to fall. When she reaches the age of forty-two, the pulse of the three [regions of] Yang deteriorates in the upper part (of the body), her entire face is wrinkled and her hair begins to turn white.

"When she reaches the age of forty-nine she can no longer become pregnant and the circulation of the great thoroughfare pulse is decreased.[7] Her menstruation is exhausted, and the gates of menstruation are no longer open; her body deteriorates and she is no longer able to bear children.

"When a boy is eight years old the emanations of his testes (kidneys 腎) are fully developed; his hair grows longer and he begins to change his teeth. When he is sixteen years of age the emanations of his testicles become abundant and he begins to secrete semen. He has an abundance of semen which he seeks to dispel; and if at this point the male and the female element unite in harmony, a child can be conceived.

"At the age of twenty-four the emanations of his testicles are regular; his muscles and bones are firm and strong, the last tooth has grown, and he has reached his full height. At thirty-two his muscles and bones are flourishing, his flesh is healthy and he is able-bodied and fertile.

6. According to the *Nan Ching*, or "Difficult Classic," chapter XXVII, *jên* (任) and *ch'ung* (衝) are two of the eight 'extraordinary' vessels which exist apart from the twelve main vessels or ducts. Hence the sentence above might also be translated: "The *jên* vessel (任 脉) begins to circulate and the *ch'ung* vessel (太 衝 脉) is (or, becomes) strong.

7. This sentence might also be translated: "The *jên* vessel becomes empty and the *ch'ung* vessel deteriorates." In the *Nan Ching*, chapter XXIX, it is said that when the *jên* vessel becomes sick it causes a stoppage of the blood in the lower abdomen (genital organs) of the woman. When the *ch'ung* vessel becomes sick it results in the formation of noxious pneuma and painful disturbances of the interior of the body which manifest themselves in a swelling of the abdomen.

"At the age of forty the emanations of his testicles become smaller, he begins to lose his hair and his teeth begin to decay. At forty-eight his masculine vigor is reduced or exhausted; wrinkles appear on his face and the hair on his temples turns white. At fifty-six the force of his liver (肝 氣) deteriorates, his muscles can no longer function properly, his secretion of semen is exhausted,[8] his vitality diminishes, his testicles (kidneys) deteriorate, and his physical strength reaches its end. At sixty-four he loses his teeth and his hair.

"Man's kidneys rule over the water which receives and stores the secretion of the five 'viscera' (五 臟)[9] and of the six 'bowels'(六 腑).[10] When the five viscera are filled abundantly, they are able to dispel secretion; but when, at this stage, the five viscera are dry, the muscles and bones decay, the generative secretions are exhausted and therefore his hair at the temples turns white, his body grows heavy, his posture is no longer straight and he is unable to produce offspring."

The Emperor asked: "But there are men who, though already old in years, produce offspring. How is this possible?"

Ch'i Po answered: "Those are men whose natural limit of age is higher. The vigor of their pulse (氣 脉) remains active and there is a surplus of secretion of their testicles (kidneys). Yet if they have children, their sons will not exceed their sixty-fourth year and their daughters will not exceed their forty-ninth year, because at that time the essence of Heaven and Earth will be exhausted."

The Emperor asked: "Those who follow Tao, the Right Way, and thus reach the age of about a hundred years, can they beget children?"

Ch'i Po answered: "Those who follow Tao, the Right Way, can escape old age and keep their body in perfect condition. Although they are old in years they are still able to produce offspring."

Huang Ti said: "I have heard that in ancient times there were the

---

8. 天 癸 (menstruation).

9. The five viscera are: heart, lungs, liver, kidneys, and stomach.

10. The six bowels are: gallbladder, stomach, large intestines, small intestines, bladder, and *San Chiao* (三 焦) the three foci. (*San Chiao*: the three foci; the three burning spaces.) "The part of the human body above the upper end of the stomach is the upper burning space (上 焦); the function of 上 焦 is to take in but not to give out. The main part of the stomach is called the middle burning space (中 焦); its function is to digest the food; (下 焦) the lower burning space is the organ of elimination; its function is to give out and not to take in." See 辭 源.

so-called Spiritual Men (真 人); they mastered the Universe and controlled Yin and Yang [the two principles in nature]. They breathed
the essence of life, they were independent in preserving their spirit,
and their muscles and flesh remained unchanged. Therefore they
could enjoy a long life, just as there is no end for Heaven and Earth.
All this was the result of their life in accordance with Tao, the
Right Way.

"In medieval times there existed the Sapients (至 人); their
virtue was preserved and they (unfailingly) upheld Tao, the Right
Way. They lived in accord with Yin and Yang, and in harmony
with the four seasons. They departed from this world and retired
from mundane affairs; they saved their energies, and preserved their
spirits completely. They roamed and travelled all over the universe
and could see and hear beyond the eight distant places. By all
these means they increased their life and strengthened it; and at
last they attained the position of the Spiritual Man.

"They were succeeded by the Sages (聖 人). The Sages attained
harmony with Heaven and Earth and followed closely the laws of
the eight winds.[11] They were able to adjust their desires to worldly
affairs, and within their hearts there was neither hatred nor anger.
They did not wish to separate their activities from the world; they
could be indifferent to custom. They did not over-exert their bodies
at physical labour and they did not over-exert their minds by strenu-
ous meditation. They were not concerned about anything, they
regarded inner happiness and peace as fundamental, and contentment as highest achievement. Their bodies could never be harmed
and their mental faculties never be dissipated. Thus they could
reach the age of one hundred years or more.

"They were succeeded by the Men of Excellent Virtue (賢 人)
who followed the rules of the universe and emulated the sun and the
moon, and they also discovered the arrangement of the stars; they
could foresee (the workings of) Yin and Yang and obey them; and

---

11. (And they follow closely the nature of the eight winds). "八 風 means: The wind
comes from eight different directions. The wind that comes from the East is called 明
庶 風 ; the wind that comes from the South-east is called 清 明 風; the wind that·
comes from the South is called 景 風; the wind that comes from the South-west is
called 涼 風; the wind that comes from the West is called 閶 闔 風; and the wind
that comes from the North-west is called 不 周 風; and the wind that comes from the
North is called 廣 莫 風; and the wind that comes from the North-east is called 融
風 *Wx.*" See: *Shuo-wên chieh-tzu* 說 文 解 字, chap. 13.

they could distinguish the four seasons. They followed the ancient times and tried to maintain their harmony with Tao. (In doing so) they increased their age toward a long·life."

2. *Great Treatise on the Harmony of the Atmosphere of the Four Seasons with the (Human) Spirit*

The three months of *Spring* are called the period of the beginning and development (of life). The breaths (氣) of Heaven and Earth are prepared to give birth; thus everything is developing and flourishing.

After a night of sleep people should get up early (in the morning); they should walk briskly around the yard; they should loosen their hair and slow down their movements (body); by these means they can (fulfill) their wish to live healthfully.

During this period (one's body) should be encouraged to live and not be killed; one should give (to it) freely and not take away (from it); one should reward (it) and not punish (it).

All this is in harmony with the breath of Spring and all this is the method for the protection of one's life.

Those who disobey the laws of Spring will be punished with an injury of the liver. For them the following Summer will bring chills and (bad) changes; thus they will have little to support their development (in Summer).

The three months of *Summer* are called the period of luxurious growth. The breaths of Heaven and Earth intermingle and are beneficial. Everything is in bloom and begins to bear fruit.

After a night of sleep people should get up early (in the morning). They should not weary during daytime and they should not allow their minds to become angry.

They should enable the best parts (of their body and spirit) to develop; they should enable their breath to communicate with the outside world; and they should act as though they loved everything outside.

All this is in harmony with the atmosphere of Summer and all this is the method for the protection of one's development.

Those who disobey the laws of Summer will be punished with an injury of the heart. For them Fall will bring intermittent fevers (痎 瘧); thus they will have little to support them for harvest (in

Fall); and hence, at Winter solstice they will suffer from grave disease.

The three months of *Fall* are called the period of tranquillity of one's conduct. The atmosphere of Heaven is quick and the atmosphere of the Earth is clear.

People should retire early at night and rise early (in the morning) with [the crowing of] the rooster. They should have their minds at peace in order to lessen the punishment of Fall. Soul and spirit should be gathered together in order to make the breath of Fall tranquil; and to keep their lungs pure they should not give vent to their desires.

All this is in harmony with the atmosphere of Fall and all this is the method for the protection of one's harvest.

Those who disobey the laws of Fall will be punished with an injury of the lungs. For them Winter will bring indigestion and diarrhoea (飧 泄); thus they will have little to support their storing (of Winter).

The three months of *Winter* are called the period of closing and storing. Water freezes and the Earth cracks open. One should not disturb one's Yang.[1]

People should retire early at night and rise late in the morning and they should wait for the rising of the sun. They should suppress and conceal their wishes, as though they had no internal purpose, as though they had been fulfilled. People should try to escape the cold and they should seek warmth, they should not perspire upon the skin, they should let themselves be deprived of breath of the cold.

All this is in harmony with the atmosphere of Winter and all this is the method for the protection of one's storing.

Those who disobey (the laws of Winter) will suffer an injury of the kidneys (testicles); for them Spring will bring impotence, and they will produce little.

The breath of Heaven is pure and light Heaven always maintains its (original) virtue; thus it never comes to fall. If Heaven opened up completely then sun and moon would never be bright, evil would come during this period of emptiness, the atmosphere of Yang would close up and the Earth would lose its brightness, clouds

1. Yang is dormant during winter. Winter is the season of Yin.

and fog would be unable to undergo changes and as a consequence
white dew would not fall, and the circulation (of the natural elements) would not communicate with the life of everything in creation.   This situation would be called "not bestowing," and as a
consequence of "not bestowing" all vegetation would perish.   Furthermore, the noxious air would not disappear, wind and rain would
not be harmonious, white dew would not fall, so that vegetation
would never again flourish.   There would always be violent winds
and sudden squalls of rain, and Heaven and Earth and the four
seasons would be unable to protect each other, they would lose Tao
and would soon be destroyed.

The sages followed the laws [of nature] and therefore their bodies
were free from strange diseases; they did not lose anything (which
they had received by nature) and their spirit of life was never
exhausted.

Those who do not conform with the breath of Spring will not
bring to life the region of the lesser Yang.   The atmosphere of their
liver will change their constitution.

Those who do not conform with the atmosphere of Summer will
not develop their greater Yang.   The atmosphere of their heart
will become empty.

Those who do not conform with the atmosphere of Fall will not
harvest their greater Yin.   The atmosphere of their lungs will be
blocked from the lower burning space.[2]

Those who do not conform with the atmosphere of Winter will
not store their lesser Yin.   The atmosphere of their testes (kidneys)
will be isolated and decreased.

Thus the interaction of the four seasons and the interaction of
Yin and Yang [the two principles in nature] is the foundation of
everything in creation.   Hence the sages conceived and developed
their Yang in Spring and Summer, and conceived and developed
their Yin in Fall and Winter in order to follow the rule of rules; and
thus [the sages], together with everything in creation, maintained
themselves at the gate of life and development.

Those who rebel against the basic rules of the universe sever their
own roots and ruin their true selves.   Yin and Yang, the two
principles in nature, and the four seasons are the beginning and the

2. Wang Ping explains: The atmosphere of the lungs cannot harvest because the lower burning space is blocked.

end of everything and they are also the cause of life and death. Those who disobey the laws of the universe will give rise to calamities and visitations, while those who follow the laws of the universe remain free from dangerous illness, for they are the ones who have obtained Tao, the Right Way.

Tao was practiced by the sages and admired by the ignorant people.[3] Obedience to the laws of Yin and Yang means life; disobedience means death. The obedient ones will rule while the rebels will be in disorder and confusion. Anything contrary to harmony (with nature) is disobedience and means rebellion to nature.

Hence the sages did not treat those who were already ill; they instructed those who were not yet ill. They did not want to rule those who were already rebellious; they guided those who were not yet rebellious. This is the meaning of the entire preceding discussion.[4] To administer medicines to diseases which have already developed and to suppress revolts which have already developed is comparable to the behavior of those persons who begin to dig a well after they have become thirsty, and of those who begin to cast weapons after they have already engaged in battle. Would these actions not be too late?

3. Wang Ping explains: Although it was admired by the ignorant people, it was not practiced by them.
4. This sentence was inserted by the commentator Wang Ping.

3. Treatise on the Communication of the Force of Life with Heaven

The Yellow Emperor said: "From earliest times the communication with Heaven has been the very foundation of life; this foundation exists between Yin and Yang and between Heaven and Earth and within the six points.[1] The (heavenly) breath prevails in the nine divisions,[2] in the nine orifices,[3] in the five viscera, and in the twelve joints; they are all pervaded by the breath of Heaven.

"Life has (the number) five, breath has (the number) three.[4]

1. The six points are: the four points of the compass, the Zenith and the Nadir.
2. These are the nine divisions of China (九 州) established under Yü the Great.
3. The nine orifices of the body: the eyes, the ears, the nostrils and the mouth, corresponding to the male principle, and the two lower orifices, the anus and the urethra, corresponding to the female principle.
4. According to Wang Ping, the three factors are: the heavenly climate, the subtle spirit of the earth, and good fortune.

If people act contrary to these factors, then noxious influences will injure mankind. This (good conduct) is the foundation of long life. Just as the breath of the blue sky (is calm), so the will and the heart of those who are pure will be in peace, and the breath of Yang will be stable in those who keep themselves in harmony with nature. Even if there are noxious spirits they cannot cause injury to those who follow the laws of the seasons. Therefore the sages preserved the natural spirit and were in harmony with the breath of Heaven, and were thus in direct communication with Heaven.

"Those who fail to preserve this (communication) will have their nine orifices closed from the inside, and the development of their muscles and flesh will be obstructed from the outside, and the breath of protection will be lost to them. This then is called: 'to injure one's own body and to destroy one's own force of life.'

"The atmosphere of Yang is similar to Heaven and to the Sun. Those who lose this (atmosphere) shorten their lives and do not prolong it. The movements of Heaven are illuminated by the sun. Yang rises up to protect man's body externally.

"In time of the cold (of winter) one should act as though one were moving around a pivot,[5] and if one behaves (moves and rests) as though one were startled, then one's spirit and breath of life will be unstable.

"In the time of the heat (of summer), if perspiration is vexatious (irregular), people pant noisily, but when they quiet down they become loquacious (confused). Then their body resembles burning charcoal and the (sickness) can be dispersed only through perspiration.

"In times of humidity (of fall) people feel as though their heads were closely bandaged, the heat of the body is expelled, and consequently the great muscles contract, while the small muscles become slack and elongated. Contraction causes cramps, slackening and elongation causes paralysis.

"In times of (hot and humid) vapors swelling occurs and the four uniting elements of the body[6] suffer successively and exhaust the atmosphere (force) of Yang. When the force of Yang is exhausted

5. The character 樞 may also be a mistake and might be read as 柩; then the sentence should read: "As though one were transporting a coffin, containing a corpse." (I.e., one should move very quietly.)
6. Wang Ping explains the uniting elements as: the muscles, the bones, the blood, and the flesh.

under the pressure of overwork and weariness, then the essence (of the body) is cut short, the openings of the body are obstructed and the secretions are retained. This causes sickness in summer and distress. Then the people's eyes are blinded and they cannot see. Their ears are closed and they cannot hear. They feel confused as though they were in a state of complete collapse and their will weakens continuously; this (condition) cannot be halted.

"If the atmosphere of Yang is exposed to great anger, the force of life of the body is interrupted and the blood rushes upwards and causes dizziness.

"When people contract an injury of their muscles, the (muscles) become lax as though they no longer existed.

"If people perspire (only) partially, they contract a partial paralysis.

"When perspiration becomes visible and meets with humidity, there will be eruptions on the skin and a weakened condition. If one perspires while (physically) weary, one is susceptible to (evil) winds which cause eruptions of the skin; and those, if irritated, will develop into sores.

"The essence of the force of Yang protects the spirit, its gentleness protects the muscles. (If the atmosphere of Yang) cannot open and close (freely), the cold air will follow and the result will be a great deformity (hunchback). The deep pulse brings about ulcers (瘻) which are transmitted to the flesh, and the breath of the ducts will become weakened, causing a propensity towards being easily frightened and startled. If the atmosphere of the (main) ducts is not harmonious with the system of the flesh, it will cause ulcers and swellings. Then the perspiration of the animal spirit (魄) is unable to reach out, one's body will be weakened, one's force of life will be melted, the '(acupuncture) spots' will be closed, and there arise winds and intermittent fevers.

"Thus wind is the cause of a hundred diseases. When people are quiet and clear, their skin and flesh is closed and protected. Even a heavy storm, afflictions, or poison, cannot injure those people who live in accord with the natural order.

"If a sickness lasts for a long time, there is danger that it might spread, then the upper and the lower (parts of the body) cannot communicate; and even skilful physicians are then not able to help.

"If Yang accumulates excessively one will die from the (resulting) disease. If the force of Yang is blocked, the blockage should be dispelled. If one does not drain it thoroughly and guide away the rough matter, there will be destruction. The force of Yang should move outwards every day.

"At dawn the breath of man comes to life; at midday the breath of Yang is most abundant; when the sun moves toward the West Yang declines, the force of Yang becomes insubstantial and the door of the breath is then closed. For this reason (the atmosphere of Yang) should be protected against bad influences, so that they cannot give trouble to the muscles and the flesh, and one should not expose them to the dew and mist of the evening. If one acts contrary to these three divisions of time, one's body will be exhausted and weakened."

Ch'i Po said: "Yin stores up essence and prepares it to be used; Yang serves as protector against external danger and must therefore be strong. If Yin is not equal to Yang, then the pulse becomes weak and sickly and causes madness. If Yang is not equal to Yin, then the breaths which are contained in the five viscera will conflict with each other and the circulation ceases within the nine orifices. For this reason the sages caused Yin and Yang to be in harmony. They caused their muscles and pulses to be in harmony, they made their bones and their marrow strong and they caused their breath and blood to be obedient (to the law of nature), so that the internal and external organs are harmonious with each other and the evil influences can do nothing that brings harm; and the ears and the eyes are quick of hearing and clear of vision, and man's force of life remains in its original state.

"If the wind enters the body and exhausts man's breath, then his essence will be lost and the evil influences will injure his liver. If man overeats, his muscles and pulses collapse and his bowels will be injured, resulting in bleeding piles. If man drinks too much his force of life becomes obstreperous. Those who indulge in excesses of sexual intercourse injure the force of their kidneys and hurt their loins. The essential principle of Yin and Yang is to preserve the element of Yang and to make it strong. If the elements do not harmonize and unite, then it is as though spring were without autumn and as though winter were without summer. But if they do harmonize and unite this harmony is called 'the system of the sages.'[7]

7. Wang Ping explains this to be the system of the sexual relations.

"Even if one's Yang is strong, but if one does not preserve it (perfectly), then the atmosphere of Yin will be exhausted. If Yin is in a state of tranquillity and Yang is preserved perfectly, then one's spirit is in perfect order. If Yin and Yang separate, one's essence and vital force will be destroyed. If then the evening dew and the wind touch one, they will cause chills and fever. This is how one is hurt by the wind, and then the evil influences will remain in the body and create a leakage.

"If one is injured in summer by the heat, then in fall one will contract intermittent fever. If one is injured in fall through humidity, it will rise to the upper part of the body and cause a cough, and this will change into paralysis (impotence 痿 厥). If one is injured in winter through the extreme cold, he will suffer from the warm disease (瘟 病) in spring.[8] The breath of the four seasons injures the five viscera in various forms.

"That which is produced by Yin originates in the five flavors; the five organs which regulate the functions of the body[9] are injured by the five flavors. Thus, if acidity exceeds the other flavors, then the liver will be caused to produce an excess of saliva and the force of the spleen will be cut short. If salt exceeds among the flavors, the great bones become weary, the muscles and the flesh become deficient and the mind becomes despondent. If sweetness exceeds the other flavors, the breath of the heart will be [asthmatic and] full, the appearance will be black and the force of the kidneys will be unbalanced. If among the flavors bitterness exceeds the others, then the atmosphere of the spleen becomes dry and the atmosphere of the stomach becomes dense. If the pungent flavor exceeds the others, the muscles and the pulse become slack and the spirit will be injured.

"Therefore if people pay attention to the five flavors and mix them well, their bones will remain straight, their muscles will remain tender and young, their breath and blood will circulate freely, their pores will be fine in texture, and consequently, their breath and bones will be filled with the essence of life.

"If, furthermore, the people carefully follow Tao as though it were a law, theirs will be a long life."

8. "The warm disease" is one of the five types of feverish diseases enumerated in the *Nan Ching*, chapter 58.
9. These five organs and their functions are: the ears for hearing, the nose for smelling, the tongue for speaking, the eyes for seeing and the skin for feeling.

4. *Treatise on the Truth of the Golden Box*

Huang Ti asked: "There are eight winds in Heaven and there are five different kinds of winds in the arteries (veins 經); how can this be explained?"

Ch'i Po answered: "When there is evil which arises from the eight winds, the evil becomes the wind of the veins and affects the five viscera; this evil will cause sickness.

"The so-called rule of the controls of the four seasons is that Spring controls Long Summer, Long Summer controls Winter, Winter controls Summer, Summer controls Fall, and Fall controls Spring. This is the so-called control of the four seasons.

"The east wind arises in Spring; its sickness is located in the liver and there are disturbances in the throat and neck. The south wind arises in Summer; its sickness is located in the heart and there are disturbances in the chest and ribs. The west wind arises in Fall; its sickness is located in the lungs and disturbances arise at the shoulders and at the back. The north wind arises in Winter; its sickness is located in the kidneys and disturbances arise in the loins and thighs. In the center there is the earth; its sickness is located in the spleen and disturbances arise in the spine.[1]

"Thus sickness resulting from the atmosphere of Spring is located in the head. Sickness resulting from the atmosphere of Summer is located in the viscera. Sickness resulting from the atmosphere of Fall is located in the shoulders and the back; and sickness resulting from the atmosphere of Winter is located in the four members of the body.

"A sickness particular to Spring is to bleed at the nose. A sickness particular to the middle part of Summer (中 夏) is located within the chest and the ribs. A sickness particular to the Long Summer is a discharge from the cavities and a cold in the center. A sickness particular to Fall is intermittent fever. A sickness particular to Winter is paralysis (convulsions 厥).

"Thus in Winter people should move in such a way that in Spring they will not bleed at the nose. Then people do not get sick in

1. The viscera: the liver, heart, lungs, kidneys, and spleen, are directly connected with the seasons, hence they are directly affected by the winds of the seasons. Throat and neck, chest and ribs, etc., are indirectly connected with the seasons, thus the various winds only cause disturbances.

Spring at their neck and throat, and they will not be sick in the middle of Summer in their chest and ribs, and during the Long Summer they do not get a discharge from the cavities and a cold in the center; they will not get intermittent fever in Fall, nor will they suffer from paralysis in Winter. (Food leaks out and perspiration appears.)[2]

"Essence is the foundation of the body; therefore if the essence is well retained within the viscera, the warm sickness (瘟) will not arise in Spring; if people do not perspire freely in the heat of Summer, they will get intermittent fever in Fall. These are the rules of the pulse and they apply to everybody.

"It is said that there is Yin within the Yin and that there is Yang within the Yang. Thus from early dawn until midday there prevails the Yang of Heaven which is the Yang within the Yang. From midday until twilight there prevails the Yang of Heaven which is the Yin within the Yang. From the time when night encloses the Earth until the first crowing of the cock there prevails the Yin of Heaven which is the Yin within the Yin. From the cock's crowing until early morning there prevails the Yin of Heaven which is the Yang within the Yin.

"Thus mankind should correspond to this system: the Yin and Yang of man are (arranged in the order) that on the outside there is Yang, and inside there is Yin. Yin and Yang of the human body (are arranged) that Yang is in back and Yin is within the front part. Yin and Yang of the (five) viscera and the (six) bowels are (arranged) that the viscera are Yin and the hollow organs are Yang. All of the five viscera, liver, heart, spleen, lungs and kidneys, are Yin; and all of the five hollow organs, gall-bladder, stomach, lower intestines, bladder, and the three burning spaces, are all Yang.

"The reason why we must know (the rule of) the Yin within the Yin and (the rule of) the Yang within the Yang is that the diseases of Winter are located in (the region of) Yang and the diseases of Summer in (the region of) Yin; the diseases of Spring are located in (the region of) Yin and the diseases of Fall in (the region of) Yang. We must know the location of all these diseases for (the purpose of) acupuncture.

"Thus the back is the (region of) Yang; the Yang within the

2. Hsin Chia Ching is in doubt about the correctness of the last sentence.

Yang is the heart. The back is the (region of) Yang and the Yin within the Yang are the lungs. The front is the (region of) Yin and the Yin within the Yin are the kidneys. The front is the (region of) Yin, and the Yang within the Yin is the liver. The front is the (region of) Yin and the extreme Yin is the spleen.

"All this is so (arranged) that Yin and Yang (complement each other) in front and back, inside and outside, as female and male element, and that they serve and respond to each other in order to conform with the Yin and Yang of Heaven."

Huang Ti asked: "Since the five viscera correspond with the four seasons, does each of the viscera receive some influence?"

Ch'i Po replied: "Yes. Green is the color of the East, it pervades the liver and lays open the eyes and retains the essential substances within the liver. Its sickness is a nervous disease, its taste is sour; its kind (element) is grass and trees (wood); its animal is the chicken; its grain is wheat; it conforms to the four seasons and corresponds to the planet Jupiter, the year star. Thus the breath of Spring is located in the head. Its sound is *chio* (角); its number is eight; and thus it becomes known that its diseases are located in the muscles; its smell is offensive and fetid.

"Red is the color of the South, it pervades the heart and lays open the ears and retains the essential substances within the heart. Its sickness is located in the five viscera; its taste is bitter; its kind (element) is fire; its animal are sheep; its grain is glutinous panicled millet; it conforms to the four seasons and corresponds to the planet Mars. And thus it becomes known that its diseases are located in the pulse; its sound is *chih* (徵); its number is seven; and its smell is scorched.

"Yellow is the color of the center; it pervades the spleen and lays open the mouth and retains the essential substances within the spleen. Its sickness is located at the root of the tongue; its taste is sweet; its kind (element) is the earth; its animal is the ox; its grain is panicled millet; it conforms to the four seasons and its star is the planet Saturn. And thus it becomes known that the disease is located within the flesh; its sound is *kung* (宮); its number is five; and its smell is fragrant and sweet.

"White is the color of the West, it pervades the lungs and lays open the nose and retains the essential substances within the lungs.

Its sickness is located within the back; its taste is pungent; its kind (element) is metal; its animals are horses; its grain is rice; it conforms to the four seasons and corresponds to Venus, the evening star. And thus it becomes known that its diseases are located in the skin and the hair; its sound is *shang* (商); its number is nine; and its smell is foul and putrid.

"Black is the color of the North, it pervades the kidneys and lays open the two lower orifices [which belong to Yin] and retains the essential substances within the kidneys. Its sickness is located within the cavities; its taste is salty; its kind (element) is water; its animals are pigs; its grain is the bean; it conforms to the four seasons and corresponds to the morning star. And thus it becomes known that its disease is located within the bones; its sound is *yü* (羽); its number is six; and its smell is rotten and evil.

"Hence the person who is adept in the investigation of the pulse should examine carefully the order of the five viscera and the six hollow organs (bowels), in regard to conformity and opposition, in regard to Yin and Yang, in regard to outside and inside, and in regard to the female and the male element; and he should keep it in mind and bring it into accord with his (superior) spirit. Not to teach it to the wrong person and never to tell or act a lie is called the achievement of Tao."

Book 2

5. *The Great Treatise on the Interaction of Yin and Yang*

THE Yellow Emperor said: "The principle of Yin and Yang [the male and female elements in nature] is the basic principle of the entire universe. It is the principle of everything in creation. It brings about the transformation to parenthood; it is the root and source of life and death; and it is also found within the temples of the gods.

"In order to treat and cure diseases one must search into their origin.

"Heaven was created by an accumulation of Yang, the element of light; Earth was created by an accumulation of Yin, the element of darkness.

"Yang stands for peace and serenity, Yin stands for recklessness and turmoil. Yang stands for destruction and Yin stands for conservation. Yang causes evaporation and Yin gives shape to things.

"Extreme cold brings forth intense heat (fever) and intense heat brings forth extreme cold (chills). Cold air generates mud and corruption; hot air generates clarity and honesty.

"If the air upon earth is clear, then food is produced and eaten at leisure. If the air above is foul, it causes dropsical swellings.

"Through these interactions of their functions, Yin and Yang, the negative and positive principles in nature, are responsible for diseases which befall those who are rebellious to the laws of nature as well as those who conform to them.

"The pure and lucid element of light represents Heaven and the turbid element of darkness represents Earth. When the vapors of the earth ascend they create clouds, and when the vapors of Heaven descend they create rain. Thus rain appears to be the climate of the earth and clouds appear to be the climate of Heaven.

"The pure and lucid element of light is manifest in the upper orifices[1] and the turbid element of darkness is manifest in the lower orifices.[2]

1. Upper orifices: mouth, ears, eyes, nostrils.
2. The two lower orifices correspond to Yin; they are the rectum and the urethral opening.

"Yang, the element of light, originates in the pores. Yin, the element of darkness, moves within the five viscera.

"Yang, the lucid element of life, is truly represented by the four extremities; and Yang, the turbid element of darkness, restores the power of the six treasuries of nature.

"Water represents Yin, and fire represents Yang. Yang creates the air and Yin creates the flavors. The flavors belong to the physical body. When the body dies the ethereal spirit is restored to the air, having thus undergone a complete metamorphosis (having thus become naturalized 歸 化).

"The ethereal spirit receives its nourishment from the air and the body receives its nourishment from the flavors.

"The ethereal spirit is created through metamorphosis, the physical shape assumes life through breath. Through transformation the ethereal spirit becomes air, and air is injurious to the perception of flavors.

"The flavors which are controlled by Yin emanate from the lower orifices. The breath (air) which is controlled by Yang emanates from the upper orifices.

"When the flavors are heavy, then Yin, the female element, is weakened and allows Yang, the male element, to enter into Yin. When the air (breath) is thick and heavy, then Yang, the male element, is reduced and allows Yin to enter into Yang.

"The heavy flavor (of the female element) then leaks out and extends itself and communicates with the aura (air) (of the male element). If this aura is thin it tends to leak out, if it is thick it becomes heated and inflamed.

"Strong passions reduce and exhaust the emanations, whereas moderate passion strengthens the emanations and makes them fertile. Strong passion consumes its emanations, whereas the emanations feed a moderate flame of lust. Strong passion scatters its emanations, whereas a moderate flame of lust begets life through its emanations.

"The pungent and the sweet flavors have a dispersing quality like Yang, the male element. The sour and the salty flavors circulate and flow like Yin, the female element.

"If Yin is healthy then Yang is apt to be defective, if Yang is healthy then Yin is apt to be sick. If the male element is victorious then there will be heat, if the female element is victorious there will be cold.

"(Exposure to) repeated and severe cold will cause (a) hot fever (sensation). Exposure to repeated and severe heat will cause a cold sensation (chills).

"Cold injures the body while heat injures the spirit.

"When the spirit is hurt severe pains ensue, when the body is hurt there will be swellings. Thus in those cases where severe pains are felt first and the swellings appear later, one can say that the spirit has injured the body. And in those cases where swellings appear first and severe pains are felt later, one can say that the body has injured the spirit.

"When wind is victorious everything moves and stirs. When the heat overcomes the world then, in the end, swellings will ensue. When dryness overcomes the world everything will be scorched. When the cold overcomes the world then everything becomes light and floating. When dampness overcomes the world then moisture will be dispelled.

"Nature has four seasons and five elements.[3] In order to grant a long life the four seasons and the five elements store up the power of creation within cold, heat, excessive dryness, moisture, and wind.

"Man has five viscera[4] in which these five climates are transformed to create joy, anger, sympathy, grief, and fear.

"The emotions of joy and anger are injurious to the spirit. Cold and heat are injurious to the body. Violent anger is hurtful to Yin, violent joy is hurtful to Yang. When rebellious emotions rise to Heaven, the pulse expires and leaves the body.

"When joy and anger are without moderation, then cold and heat exceed all measure and life is no longer secure. Yin and Yang should be respected to an equal extent.

"It is said: When people are injured through the severe cold of Winter, the sickness will recur in Spring. When people are hurt through the wind in Spring, they will not be able to retain their food in Summer. When people are hurt through the extreme heat of Summer, they will get intermittent fever in Fall. When people are hurt through the humidity of Fall, they will get a cough in Winter."

The Yellow Emperor said: "It is said that in former times the

3. Metal, wood, water, fire, and earth.
4. Liver, heart, stomach, lungs, and kidneys.

ancient sages discoursed on the human body and that they enumerated separately each of the viscera and each of the bowels. They
talked about the origin of the blood vessels and about the vascular
system, and said that where the blood vessels and the arteries (veins)
meet there are six junctions. Following the course of each of the
arteries there are the (365) vital points for acupuncture.

"Each of these points has a place and a name, just as 'hollow'
refers to the bones, and they all have sections which set them apart
from each other.

"No matter whether people are rebellious or obedient there is
method and regularity in the workings of the four seasons and Yin
and Yang. Everything is subject to their invariable rules and regulations, which govern the relationship between external and internal
influences. Are there not also internal and external symptoms (of
diseases)?"

Ch'i Po answered: "The East creates the wind; wind creates
wood; wood creates the sour flavor; the sour flavor strengthens the
liver; the liver nourishes the muscles; the muscles strengthen the
heart; and the liver governs the eyes. The eyes see the darkness
and mystery of Heaven and they discover Tao, the Right Way,
among mankind.

"Upon earth there is transformation and change which produce
the five flavors. The attainment of Tao (the Right Way) produces
wisdom, while the supernatural [powers] (神) spring from darkness
and mystery.

"The supernatural [powers] create wind in Heaven and they
create wood upon earth. Within the body they create muscles and
of the five viscera they create the liver. Of the colors they create
the green color and of the musical notes they create the note *chio*
(角); and they give to the human voice the ability to form a shouting
sound. In times of excitement and change they grant the capacity
for control. Of the orifices they create the eyes, of the flavors they
create the sour flavor, and of the emotions they create anger.

"Anger is injurious to the liver, but sympathy counteracts anger.
Wind is injurious to the muscles, but heat and drought counteract
the wind. The sour flavor is injurious to the muscles, but the
pungent flavor counteracts the sour flavor.

"From the South there comes extreme heat. Heat produces fire
and fire produces the bitter flavor. The bitter flavor strengthens

the heart, the heart nourishes the blood and the blood enlivens the stomach.   The heart rules over the tongue.

"The supernatural [powers] (神) of Summer create heat in Heaven and fire upon Earth.   They create the pulse within the body and the heat within the viscera.   Of the colors they create the red color and of the musical notes they create *chih* (徵) and they give to the human voice the ability to express joy.   In times of excitement and change they grant the capacity for sadness and grief.   Of the orifices they create the mouth with its palate; of the flavors they create the bitter flavor, and of the emotions they create happiness and joy.

"Extravagant joy is injurious to the heart, but fear counteracts happiness.   Heat is injurious to the spirit, but the cold of Winter counteracts the heat of Summer.   The bitter flavor is injurious to the spirit, but the salty flavor counteracts the bitter flavor.

"Humidity is created by the center.   Humidity nourishes the earth and the earth produces sweet flavors.   The sweet flavor nourishes the stomach, the stomach strengthens the flesh, and the flesh protects the lungs.   The stomach rules over the mouth.

"The [mysterious] powers of the earth create humidity in Heaven and fertile soil upon earth.   They create the flesh within the body, and of the viscera they create the stomach.   Of the colors they create the yellow color, and of the musical notes they create the note *kung* (宮), and they give to the human voice the ability to sing.   In times of excitement and change they cause the emission of belching.[5] Of the orifices they create the mouth, of the flavors they create the sweet flavor, and of the emotions they create consideration and sympathy.

"Extreme sympathy is injurious to the stomach, but anger counteracts sympathy.   Humidity is injurious to the flesh, but wind counteracts humidity.   The sweet flavor hurts the flesh, but the sour flavor counteracts the sweet flavor.

"Scorched dryness is created by the West.   Dryness creates metal and metal produces the pungent flavor.   The pungent flavor nourishes the lungs and the lungs strengthen the skin and the hair.   Skin and hair protect the kidneys.   The lungs govern the nose.

"The [mysterious] powers of Fall create dryness in Heaven and they create metal upon Earth.   Upon the body they create skin and hair, and of the viscera they create the lungs.   Of the colors

5. Wang Ping equals 噦 (to belch), to 噦 氣 忤 (to be obstinate).

they create the white color, and of the musical notes they create *shang* (商), and they give to the human voice the ability to weep and to wail. In times of excitement and change they create a cough. Of the orifices they create the nose with its nostrils, among the flavors they create the pungent flavor, and among the emotions they create grief.

"Extreme grief is injurious to the lungs, but joy counteracts grief. Heat is injurious to skin and hair, but cold temperature counteracts heat. The pungent flavor is injurious to skin and hair, but the bitter flavor counteracts the pungent flavor.

"Extreme cold is created in the north. Cold creates water, and water creates salt. Salt nourishes the kidneys and the kidneys strengthen the bones and the marrow; and the marrow strengthens the liver. The kidneys rule over the ears.

"The [mysterious] powers of Winter create the extreme cold in Heaven and they create water upon earth. Within the body they create the bones, and of the orifices they create the kidneys (testicles). Of the colors they create the black color, and of the musical notes they create the note *yü* (羽). They give to the human voice the ability to groan and to hum. In times of excitement and change they create trembling, and among the emotions they create fear.

"Extreme fear is injurious to the kidneys, but fear can be overcome by contemplation. The cold is injurious to the blood, but dry heat counteracts the cold. Salt is injurious to the blood, but the sweet flavor counteracts salt.

"Hence it is said: Heaven and Earth are the highest and lowest of all creation. Yin and Yang [the two elements in nature] create desires and vigor in men and women. The ways of Yin and Yang are to the left and to the right. Water and fire are the evidences and symbols of Yin and Yang. Yin and Yang are the source of power and the beginning of everything in creation.

"Hence it is said: Yin is active within and acts as guardian of Yang; Yang is active on the outside and acts as regulator of Yin."

The Yellow Emperor asked: "Is there any alternative to the laws of Yin and Yang?"

Ch'i Po answered: "When Yang is stronger the body is hot, the pores are closed and the people begin to pant; they become boisterous and coarse and whether one looks up or down no perspiration appears. People become feverish (hot), their gums are dry and give

trouble, the stomach is affected (oppressed) and people die of constipation. When Yang is stronger people can endure Winter but they
cannot endure Summer.

"When Yin is stronger the body is cold and perspiration appears
regularly all over the body. People see their fate clearly; they
tremble with fear and get chilled. When they are chilled their
spirits become rebellious. Their full stomachs can no longer digest
and they die. When Yin is stronger people can endure Summer but
they cannot endure Winter.

"Thus Yin and Yang alternate, their victories vary and so does
the character of their diseases."

The Yellow Emperor asked: "Can anything be done to blend and
to adjust these two principles in nature?"

Ch'i Po answered: "If one has the ability to know the seven injuries and the eight advantages, the two principles can be brought
into harmony. If one does not know how to use this knowledge then
his span of life will be limited by early decay.

"At the age of forty the Yin element within the body is reduced
to one half of its natural capacity and man's usual behaviour
deteriorates.

"At the age of fifty the body grows heavy and the ears no longer
hear well nor is the vision of the eyes clear any longer.

"At the age of sixty the life-producing force of Yin declines and
impotence sets in. The nine orifices no longer benefit each other.
The orifices below become insubstantial and vacant while those
above remain substantial and real, and the ability to weep is totally
exhausted.

"Yet it is said: Those who have the true wisdom remain strong
while those who have no knowledge and wisdom grow old and feeble.
Therefore the people should share this wisdom and their names will
become famous. Those who are wise inquire and search together,
while those who are ignorant and stupid inquire and search apart
from each other. Those who are stupid and ignorant do not exert
themselves enough in the search for the Right Way, while those who
are wise search beyond the natural limits.

"Those who search beyond the natural limits will retain good
hearing and clear vision, their bodies will remain light and strong,
and although they grow old in years they will remain able-bodied
and flourishing; and those who are able-bodied can govern to great
advantage.

"For this reason the ancient sages practiced (爲 無 爲) not to undertake any worldly affairs, and in their pleasures and joys they ere dignified and tranquil. They followed their own desires and they never directed their will and ambition toward the protection of a purpose that was empty of meaning. Thus their allotted span of life was without limit, like Heaven and Earth. This was the way the ancient sages controlled and conducted themselves.

"Heaven is not complete with only the West and the North; the West and the North are the regions of Yin. Man's hearing and eyesight are not so clear on his right side as they are on his left side.[6]

"The Earth is not complete with only the East and the South; the East and the South are the regions of Yang. Man's left hand and foot are not so strong as are his right hand and foot."[7]

The Yellow Emperor asked: "How is this possible?"

Ch'i Po answered: "The East is the region of Yang, the element of light. The essences of Yang unite and ascend to Heaven, thus there is clarity and light above and darkness and unreality below. This causes excellent hearing and clear vision, whereas hands and feet cannot be used to advantage.

"The West is the region of Yin, the element of darkness. The essences of Yin unite and descend to the earth; thus there is abundance and clarity below, while everything above is empty and unreal. This causes hearing and eyesight to be impaired, whereas hands and feet can be employed to advantage.

"Everything can be influenced by harmful emanations. When they ascend, the right becomes more affected; when they descend, the left side becomes affected. Thus neither Heaven and Earth, nor Yin and Yang—nothing can be complete because of the existence of these harmful emanations.

"In Heaven there are ethereal spirits; upon earth there is form and shape. In Heaven there are eight regulators;[8] upon earth there are five principles;[9] and by means of these all living creatures can be transformed into parents.

"Yang, the lucid element, ascends to Heaven. Yin, the turbid element, returns to earth. Hence the Universe (Heaven and Earth)

6. *Yu*, the right side, also indicates the West.
7. *Tso*, the left side, also indicates the East.
8. Wang Ping equals the eight regulators to the eight winds.
9. Wang Ping equals 五 里, the five ways or principles, to 五 行, the five elements.

represents motion and rest, controlled by the wisdom of nature (the gods). Nature grants the power to beget and to grow, to harvest and to store, to finish and to begin anew.

"The Men of Virtue (賢 人) matched Heaven when they cultivated their minds; they resembled the Earth when they provided sufficient nourishment; and they were by the side of the people in the care of the five viscera.

"The heavenly climate circulates within the lungs; the climate of the earth circulates within the throat; the wind circulates within the liver, thunder penetrates the heart; the air of a ravine penetrates the stomach; the rain penetrates the kidneys. The six arteries generate streams; the bowels and the stomach generate the oceans; the nine orifices generate flowing water; and Heaven and Earth generate Yin and Yang [the two opposing principles].

"The perspiration which is generated by Yang is of the same importance as the rain which is generated by the Universe. The air which is generated by Yang is of the same importance as the strong wind which is generated by the Universe. Violent behaviour and scorching air resemble thunder. Rebellious behaviour resembles Yang.

"Regulation and treatment without method show that the rules of Heaven are not being followed, and calamities and visitations upon earth will reach their utmost.

"Evil customs affect the body as much as wind and rain affect the body.

"Those who give their bodies a good cure (first) treat their skin and hair; their next treatment concerns itself with the muscles and the flesh; the treatment after that concerns itself with the six bowels; and the next treatment concerns itself with the five viscera. The treatment of the five viscera should take place halfway between life and death.

"When Heaven is affected by noxious emanations, then man's five viscera receive injuries. When water and grain are affected by cold or heat, then man's six bowels receive injuries. When the earth is affected by humidity, then man's skin, flesh, muscles and pulse receive injuries.

"Those who are experts in using the needle for acupuncture follow Yin, the female principle, in order to draw out Yang. And they follow Yang, the male principle, in order to draw out Yin. They use the right hand in order to treat the illness of the left side, and they use the left hand in order to treat the illness of the right side.

"By observing myself I know about others and their diseases are revealed to me, and by observing the external symptoms one gathers knowledge about internal disturbances. One should watch beyond the ordinary limits for rules which are unfit and inadequate; one should observe minute and trifling things as if they were of normal size, and when they are thus treated they cannot become dangerous.

"Those who are experts in examining patients judge their general appearance; they feel the pulse and distinguish whether it is Yin or Yang that causes the disease. If the appearance changes from clear to turbid, then the location of the disease is revealed. Coughing and short-windedness should be watched carefully; one should listen to the sounds and the notes and then the location of the affliction will become apparent. One should examine irregularities which must be adjusted according to custom and usage, and then the location where the disease prevails will become known.

"One should feel the pulse at the place of the 'cubit' (尺) and at the place of the 'inch' (寸) and one should observe whether the pulse is superficial or whether it is deep, whether it is regular or uneven; and then it becomes evident where the disease originates and it can be cured.

"Nothing surpasses the examination of the pulse, for with it errors cannot be committed. Therefore it is said: the disease can be brought to decline. For, although a disease may be light it can nevertheless spread; and although a disease may be grave it can nevertheless be improved; and by the time the disease has disappeared completely it has also become well-known.

"If material things are not able to revive a patient, breath must be used; and if the spiritual essence is not able to bring improvement to a patient, the five flavors must be applied. The gravest illness can thus be overcome and the lightest illness can thus be brought to decline and finally be exhausted.

"Those who are completely affected (中 滿) can then be brought to dispel it within, and those who are possessed by evil influences cleanse their bodies through perspiration. When the disease is located at the skin it will become manifest through perspiration.

"When the pulse of those who are afraid and trembling and of those who are cruel and violent is felt, it will contract. When the pulse is full, long and slightly tense, the disease will be dissolved and the patients relieved from disease.

"In order to examine whether Yin or Yang predominates one must distinguish a gentle pulse and one of low tension from a hard and bounding pulse.[10] During a disease of Yang, Yin predominates; and during a disease of Yin, Yang predominates. When vigor and constitution are determined everything is in its proper place.

"When the blood hardens it should be cleared and made to burst forth. When the breath fades that part which obstructs the breath should be stretched."

10. Wang Ping says: A Yang-pulse is strong and bounding while a Yin-pulse is weak and of low tension.

6. Treatise on the Parting and Meeting of Yin and Yang

The Yellow Emperor said: "It is said that Heaven was created by Yang (the male principle of light and life), and that the Earth was created by Yin (the female principle of darkness and death). It is said that the sun represents Yang, and that the moon represents Yin. The large and the small months[1] added together resulted in three hundred and sixty days and this made one year, and mankind always lived in accord with this system. Is it true that nowadays the three elements of Yang no longer correspond with the system of Yin and Yang of old?"

Ch'i Po answered: "Yin and Yang may be added up to amount to the number ten; this can be extended and may mean one hundred; or the number may be estimated to be one thousand and this can be extended and mean ten thousand, that is to say: it includes everything. Ten thousand is so large that it cannot be matched by any number, and the same is true of its importance.

"Everything in creation is covered by Heaven and supported by the Earth; when nothing has as yet come forth (been grown, produced) the Earth is called: the place where Yin dwells; it is also known as the Yin within the Yin. Yang supplies that which is upright, while Yin, the Earth, acts as a ruler of Yang.

"Planting and begetting are in accord with Spring; growing and

1. 月 大 , a large month of thirty days in the lunar calendar; 月 小, a small month of twenty-nine days in the lunar calendar.

cultivating are in accord with Summer; gathering in the harvest is in accord with Fall, and the storing of the crop is in accord with Winter. If people habitually neglect to follow these rules, then the work of Heaven and Earth and of the four seasons will be impeded. If Yin and Yang change the people will change likewise, and their destiny can then be prefigured."

The Yellow Emperor said: "I should like to hear more about the parting and meeting of Yin and Yang."

Ch'i Po answered: "The ancient sages faced the South and thus they established themselves. Whatever was before them was spoken of as shining space(廣 明), and whatever was behind them was called the great thoroughfare or the Great Yang.

"The Great Yang is located within the soil and in it is the lesser Yin. When this lesser Yin rises above the Earth, it comes under the influence of the Great Yang.

"The Great Yang is the foundation of existence from the beginning to the end. The Great Yin is the connecting link between life and the 'Gate of Life'[2] (命 門), and thus it becomes evident that within the Yin there is also a Yang. It is within the body and above and it is called shining space; but if this shining expanse sends its rays below then it is spoken of as the great Yin. The front of the Great Yin is known to be illuminated by the 'sunlight'.

"The 'sunlight' is the foundation of everything, it permeates everything and it is therefore known as the Yang within the Yin. If Yin becomes apparent externally then it is known as the lesser Yang.

"The lesser Yang is the foundation of and brings to life the orifices of Yin, and hence it is called the lesser Yang within the Yin.

"This then is the parting and the meeting of the three Yang. The Great Yang acts as opening factor, the 'sunlight' acts as covering factor, and the lesser Yang acts as axis or central point.

"The three main arteries (經) must not miss each other; they must be drawn together and when their pulse does not sound superficial then its name is one Yang (pulse)."

The Yellow Emperor said: "I should like to know more about the three Yin."

---

2. The 'Gate of Life' is supposed to be located between the kidneys and is held to be the organ where the blood undergoes the transformation into semen.

Ch'i Po answered: "On the outside there is Yang but within it is Yin that is active.   Yin is active in the interior and is effective below; there its name is the great Yin.

"The great Yin is the foundation of everything that is hidden, mysterious, and empty; and thus it is called the Yin within the Yin. The rear of the Great Yin is called the lesser Yin (少 陰).

"The lesser Yin is the origin of all that flows rapidly and of all the springs, and it is spoken of as the lesser Yin within the Yin.

"The front of the lesser Yin is called the 'absolute Yin'.   This Yin is the foundation of greatness and honesty.   Where Yin breaks off there is Yang, and at that point it is called the Yin within the absolute Yin.

"Here we have the parting and the meeting of the three Yin.   The great Yin acts as opening factor, the absolute Yin acts as covering factor, and the lesser Yin acts as axis or central point.

"The three main arteries must not miss each other; they must be drawn together, and when their pulse does not sound deep then it is called one Yin (pulse).

"The climates of Yin and Yang alternate and their accumulated climates act as one complete unit.   The internal spirit and the external physical shape perfect each other."

7. *Treatise on Yin and Yang Treated Separately*

The Yellow Emperor said: "Man has four main arteries and twelve subsidiary vessels."[1]

Ch'i Po answered: "The four main arteries correspond to the four seasons, the twelve vessels correspond to the twelve months, and the twelve months correspond to the twelve pulses.

"The pulses consist of Yin and Yang, the two principles in nature. When the proportion of Yang is known Yin is revealed; and when the proportion of Yin is known Yang is revealed.   The five viscera are permeated by the Yang element, and each of the five viscera has five Yang elements; thus there are five times five, or twenty-five Yang elements.   Of the intestines some belong entirely to the Yin element,[2] and when these become visible they become impaired; and when these intestines are impaired death follows.   Some of the

1. The vascular system consists of twelve pairs of main vessels and their respective branches. They carry the blood and the air to different parts of the body.
2. The solid organs.

intestines belong entirely to the Yang element, and those are the ducts in the body and the stomach.

"When Yang is treated separately then the location of the disease will be revealed; and when Yin is treated separately then the expectancy of life and the date of death are revealed.

"The three Yang (pulses) are located in the head and the three Yin (pulses) are located in the hand; and together they form one entity.

"When Yang is treated separately it becomes known what disease should be feared in what season; when Yin is treated separately the dates of life and death become known. If one is attentive to the laws of Yin and Yang, one does not plan with these two principles as though they were one whole.

"It is said about Yin and Yang that those who kill are influenced by Yin, those who reach the highest good are influenced by Yang; those who are peaceful and quiet are influenced by Yin, and those who are active are influenced by Yang; those who are slow and dilatory are influenced by Yin, and those who are quick are influenced by Yang.

"In general it can be said that life is supported by the true pulse of the viscera. When the pulse of the liver is extremely uneven and hasty, death ensues after eighteen days; when the pulse of the heart is extremely uneven, death ensues after nine days; when the pulse of the lungs is very uneven, death ensues after twelve days; when the pulse of the kidneys is very uneven, death ensues after seven days; when the pulse of the spleen is very uneven, death ensues after four days.

"The disease of the two Yang[3] affects the heart and the spleen, and this must not remain hidden and ignored; otherwise woman will not menstruate and man will not have a sufficient monthly emanation. If this disease is perpetuated, then it has a destructive and dissipating influence which—if spread—inhibits all energies; and death cannot be warded off.

"It is said that the three Yang[4] cause diseases whereby chills or fevers are produced, and these diseases cause ulcers and swellings within the body; these ultimately lead to impotence, hiccoughing, heavy breathing, and contusions.

3. Wang Ping equals "two Yang" to the 'sunlight' and the 'great Yang.'
4. Wang Ping equals "three Yang" to the 'great Yin,' the 'sunlight' and the 'lesser Yang.'

"When these diseases spread they cause exhaustion and dampness, and transmitted they cause decay and hernia.

"It is said that one element of Yang causes shortness of breath and makes the people susceptible to coughing and diarrhoea. When these diseases are spread they cause a throbbing of the heart, and when perpetuated cause irregularity (of the bodily functions).

"Two elements of Yang plus one element of Yin produce diseases indicated by alarm and terror; the back aches, people are apt to belch and to be deficient in strength. The name of this disease is: wind and convulsions.

"Two elements of Yin and one element of Yang create a disease which causes swellings, and the heart is filled with vapors.

"Three elements of Yang and three elements of Yin cause a disease which produces paralysis on one side and various transformations, so that the four limbs cannot be raised and moved.

"When one element of Yang is aroused it is called a 'hook' (鈎); when one element of Yin is aroused it is called a 'hair' (毛). The Yang which has to be aroused to overcome acute trouble is taut like a tremulous musical string (絃). To arouse Yang to its utmost and then to break off is called a 'stone' (石). When Yin and Yang flow together it is called 'a stream' (溜).

"Yin strives towards the interior; Yang reaches towards the outside, taking the shape of perspiration which cannot be concealed. Disobedience to the four seasons will surely manifest itself, and this manifestation will take the shape of an evil disease of the lungs, causing the people to pant and to breathe with difficulty.

"Yin creates peace and harmony; and the root of everything is peace and harmony. Hence when this state is constant it yields endurance. The emanations of Yang have a dispersing and destructive effect.

"Peace consists of hard and soft particles; it is not uniform and enduring, and its life-giving principle can be interrupted.

"When death is brought about by (a disease of) Yin, it will take but three days for death to occur; and life, produced by Yang (alone), lasts but four days and then death occurs. This is the so-called life when it is connected with Yang; and death when it is connected with Yin.

"When the liver strengthens the heart, we speak of life supported by Yang. When the heart nourishes the liver, we speak of death as connected with Yin. When the lungs strengthen the kidneys, we speak of the importance of Yin. When the kidneys strengthen the spleen we speak of the punishment of Yin; and death cannot be averted.

"When Yang coagulates the four limbs swell up. When Yin coagulates it is advantageous to draw one pint[5] of blood; when it coagulates twice two pints should be drawn; when it coagulates three times, three pints should be drawn. When Yin and Yang congeal then the situation is oblique. (The situation when there are) too many elements of Yin and too few elements of Yang is called 'barren.'

"When there is not enough water the stomach swells. When two elements of Yang[6] connect the result is digestion. When three elements of Yang[7] connect the result is a filtering system. The effect of the connection of three elements of Yin[8] is called 'water.'

"When one element of Yin and one element of Yang[9] connect, the effect is called numbness of the throat. When Yin attacks and Yang separates, it is said that a child has been conceived. When Yin and Yang are hollow and empty, the bowels are washed out and death ensues. When Yang equals Yin it becomes apparent through perspiration. When Yin is empty and hollow and Yang is full and abundant,[10] the result is called a 'collapse' (menorrhagia).

"When the three Yin[11] attack and rush toward each other death will ensue at midnight after twenty days. When two elements of Yin[12] attack, death will occur after thirteen days at dusk. When three elements of Yang attack, everything swells and death ensues

5. 升 *shêng*, a pint, a measure equivalent to 3⅓ cubic inches.
6. Wang Ping equals the two elements of Yang to the stomach plus the lower intestines.
7. Wang Ping equals the three elements of Yang to the small intestines, the bladder and the groins.
8. Wang Ping explains: The connection of the three elements of Yin means that the pulses of the spleen and of the lungs indicate coagulation and chills. This creates a change in temperature and generates water.
9. Wang Ping explains: The connection of the pulse and the heart with the pulse of the three foci creates internal fevers.
10. Wang Ping explains: When the pulse of Yin is insufficient and the pulse of Yang abundant, then it causes internal ruin and blood flows out below.
11. Wang Ping explains: The pulses of the spleen and of the lungs have more than the necessary number of beats.
12. Wang Ping explains: The pulses of the heart and of the kidneys have more than the necessary number of beats.

after three days. When three elements of Yang and three elements of Yin attack and rush towards each other, then heart and stomach are packed full and cannot be emptied entirely of hidden and small matter, and death ensues after five days. When two elements of Yang attack, the patient's sickness will recur, death cannot be warded off, and the patient will die after ten days."

Book 3

8. *Treatise on the Ingeniousness and Subtlety of the Secret Records*

THE Yellow Emperor said: "I desire to hear how it is possible that the twelve viscera send each other that which is precious and that which is worthless."

Ch'i Po answered: "How can I best answer this question? May I ask you to follow these words: the heart is like the minister of the monarch who excels through insight and understanding; the lungs are the symbol of the interpretation and conduct of the official jurisdiction and regulation; the liver has the functions of a military leader who excels in his strategic planning; the gall bladder occupies the position of an important and upright official who excels through his decisions and judgment; the middle of the thorax (the part between the breasts) is like the official of the center who guides the subjects in their joys and pleasures; the stomach acts as the official of the public granaries and grants the five tastes; the lower intestines are like the officials who propagate the Right Way of Living, and they generate evolution and change; the small intestines are like the officials who are trusted with riches, and they create changes of the physical substance; the kidneys are like the officials who do energetic work, and they excel through their ability and cleverness; the burning spaces are like the officials who plan the construction of ditches and sluices, and they create waterways; the groins and the bladder are like the magistrates of a region[1] or a district, they store the overflow and the fluid secretions which serve to regulate vaporization. These twelve officials should not fail to assist one another.

"When the monarch is intelligent and enlightened, there is peace and contentment among his subjects; they can thus beget offspring, bring up their children, earn a living and lead a long and happy life. And because there are no more dangers and perils, the earth is considered glorious and prosperous.

"But when the monarch is not intelligent and enlightened, the twelve officials become dangerous and perilous; the use of Tao, (the

1. 州 a region, a department or political division; anciently 2500 families.

Right Way) is obstructed and blocked, and Tao no longer circulates warnings against physical excesses. When one attains Tao (the Right Way), even in small and trifling matters, the change will not exhaust and impoverish the people, for they know how to search for themselves.

"Afflicted are those who dissipate; they become nervous and startled. But those who are aware of their needs and desires are encouraged, and as an expression of this encouragement they become peace-loving and virtuous.

"The number of those who are confused and dim of vision is like the number of atoms and hair. Their number can be judged to be one hundred times ten thousand, and even this can be increased; and when it is this large, its shape can be regulated."

The Yellow Emperor said: "Excellent, indeed! I have been told that Tao, the Right Way of essence and brightness, was the great calling of the Emperor and that he proclaimed and illustrated the great Tao; he warned those who were not pure and temperate, and he selected a lucky day when no one dared to inflict suffering. Now the Yellow Emperor selects a lucky day with an auspicious omen to collect the ingenious and subtle secrets and to hand them down for safekeeping."

9. *Treatise on the Six Regulations Governing the Manifestations of the Viscera*

The Yellow Emperor said: "I understand that Heaven employs six times six regulations (sections, divisions of time 節) in order to make one year, and that man needs nine times nine laws in order to form society.

"According to plan, man consists of three hundred and sixty-five parts (joints, sections) which have come to be regarded as being similar to the parts of the Universe. I am ignorant of the meaning of this."

Ch'i Po answered: "How can I illustrate this question? I beg of you to follow my words: Six times six regulations (terms, divisions of time) and nine times nine laws are combined in order to adjust the rules of nature and the corresponding destiny.

"After the rules of Heaven have thus been adjusted, sun and moon can go into action; destiny can thus be regulated (紀) and transformation and birth can begin to function.

"Heaven represents Yang and the Earth represents Yin; the sun represents Yang and the moon represents Yin. The (movement of) sun and moon share in their duties as regulators; one completed movement (revolution of the sun) serves as basic principle for Tao. The sun moves one measure while the moon moves thirteen measures and more. The large and small months make three hundred and sixty-five days and thus complete one year. Since there is a surplus of amassed atmosphere (氣), it is taken care of by inserting intercalary days and months.[1]

"In the beginning a doctrine is established; important things are placed in the middle; the surplus is pushed to the end; and thus the measure of Heaven is completed."

The Yellow Emperor said: "I have heard the law of Heaven before, now I should like to hear whether it has any relationship to human destiny."

Ch'i Po answered: "Heaven employs six times six regulations (divisions of time), and the earth uses nine times nine laws to form one whole. Heaven has ten celestial stems,[2] the day has six (pairs of horary characters)[3] which revolve. When *chia*, the first celestial stem, has returned six times, a cycle of sixty years, or one lifetime, has been completed, based on the standard of three hundred sixty days to one year.

"From olden times communication with Heaven was the origin of life; and from the beginning of time the breath of Yin and Yang, the female and the male principles in nature, circulated through the nine provinces (九 州) as well as through the nine orifices. Life is influenced by five elements, spirit is influenced by three factors. Three factors serve to complete Heaven, and three factors serve to complete the earth, and three factors serve to complete man. Three times three factors make nine, and nine acts as the nine sections (里 子), and the nine sections are the nine viscera.

"The external body has four viscera[4] and the internal body has

1. An intercalary month is inserted seven times in nineteen years to make up the deficiencies in the solar and lunar years.
2. The ten celestial stems: 甲 乙 丙 丁 戊 已 庚 辛 壬 癸.
3. The twelve horary characters: 子 丑 寅 卯 辰 巳 午 末 申 酉 戌 亥.
4. Wang Ping enumerates the four viscera of the external body: 1. head, 2. ears and eyes, 3. mouth and teeth, 4. the thorax (the mind).

five viscera;[5] and they unite, thus making nine viscera, corresponding to the general system."

The Emperor said: "I have also heard that six times six and nine times nine unite, but why is it then that the surplus of amassed atmospheric power is taken care of by inserting intercalary days and months? I should like to know about the meaning of this amassed atmospheric power, and I beg of you to lift this veil of ignorance and to dispel my doubts."

Ch'i Po answered: "That which was kept secret by the emperors of old was propagated and perpetuated by the early teachers."

The Emperor said "I beg you to continue your words."

Ch'i Po said: "Five days are called a 'period of five days';[6] three of these five-day periods are called 'one of the twenty-four solar periods of the year'; six of these solar periods are called 'one season', four seasons are called 'one year'; and each of these periods is subject to a different control.

"The interaction of the five elements brings harmony and everything is in order. At the end of one year the sun has completed its course and everything starts anew with the first season, which is the beginning of Spring.[7] This system is comparable to a ring which has neither beginning nor end. The periods of five days each also share this arrangement. Therefore I must say: those who are ignorant about the increase of the year, and about that which is produced through the flourishing, deteriorating, emptying, and filling powers of the four seasons cannot produce good work."

The Yellow Emperor said: "The interaction of the five elements is like a ring—it has no beginning; is this an excessive or inadequate description?"

Ch'i Po answered: "The five atmospheric influences[8] change their spheres of activity; they counteract one another and there is constancy in their transformation from abundance to emptiness."

The Emperor asked: "How can one achieve a tranquil atmosphere?"

5. Wang Ping enumerates the five viscera of the internal body: 1. liver, 2. heart, 3. spleen, 4. lungs, 5. kidneys.
6. 候 , a period of five days; seventy-two periods of five days make up one year. Every period had its name which gave an indication of the season; three of these periods made one *chieh* (節), and the total made one year.
7. 立 氣 = 立 春 , beginning of Spring, about February 5–18.
8. The five atmospheric influences (五 氣) are: rain which is under the influence of wood; fine weather which is under the influence of metal; heat which is under the influence of fire; cold which is under the influence of water; and wind which is under the influence of earth.

Ch'i Po answered: "By avoiding transgressions of the laws of nature."

The Emperor asked: "If this perfection cannot be achieved—what then?"

Ch'i Po answered: "This perfection is contained in the invariable rules of conduct."

The Emperor asked: "What is the meaning of counteraction?"

Ch'i Po answered: "Spring counteracts the long Summer (長 夏); the long Summer counteracts Winter; Winter counteracts Fall; Fall counteracts Spring. This is called the effect of the counteraction of the five elements and their respective seasons. Each element uses its life-giving principle to influence the destiny of its particular viscera."

The Emperor asked: "How can one use this knowledge of their counteraction?"

Ch'i Po answered: "By seeking after the highest (good). Everything is restored at the beginning of Spring.[9] If people have not yet arrived at the highest (good) but nevertheless reach out for it, their action is called 'excessive'. Then there is carelessness everywhere, which cannot be counteracted, and that which must be overcome is multiplied. General behaviour becomes immoral and licentious, and people no longer segregate those whose inner life is depraved and heterodox, and those in office cannot enforce restrictions and prohibitions.

"Those who strive for the highest (good), yet cannot attain it, are called unequal to the task. Then that which has already been gained is squandered in foolish and reckless conduct. This produces suffering of diseases because of carelessness, which cannot be overcome. At these critical times those who seek after the highest (good) turn to the highest life-giving principles of the respective season.

"Even though one attends respectfully to the periods of five days, to the seasons and their atmospheric influences, it is still possible to make mistakes in regard to the full year and to act against the system of the five-day periods and the five elements. Then one can no longer segregate oneself from those whose inner life is depraved and heterodox; and those in office can no longer enforce restrictions and prohibitions."

9. Wang Ping explains that 始 春, the beginning of Spring, is equal to 立 春, February 5-18, one of the twenty-four solar terms.

The Emperor asked: "Is there no hereditary influence?"

Ch'i Po answered: "The atmospheric influence of the blue sky is constant, but this climate cannot be inherited and it is called 'extraordinary and unusual.' Because it is extraordinary it changes (while Heaven remains constant and invariable)."[10]

The Emperor asked: "How can it be extraordinary and yet change?"

Ch'i Po answered: "The change affects the body and thus brings disease. If this disease can be overcome it remains invisible and trifling, if it cannot be overcome it will become more important than its cause and very severe; and if evil influences are added death will ensue. Thus if one acts wrong in regard to the seasons his action may remain secret and hidden, but if one follows the laws of the seasons he will be considered great."

The Emperor said: "Excellent indeed! I have also heard that the atmospheric influences unite and take shape, and because of this change one can define them in precise terms. The revolution of Heaven and Earth and the transformations brought about by Yin and Yang have their effect upon everything in creation. Can we also obtain knowledge about the extent of this influence?"

Ch'i Po said: "How brilliant a question! Heaven is boundless and cannot be measured. The Earth is large and without limit. In order to find out how large one must ask Ling Shên[11] and beg him for information on the extent of those regions.

"Grass and herbs bring forth the five colors;[12] nothing that can be seen excels the variation of these five colors. Grass and herbs also produce the five flavors;[13] nothing excels the deliciousness of these five flavors. Human desires are not alike, therefore everyone has at his disposal all of them.

"Man receives the five atmospheric influences as food from Heaven and the five flavors as food from Earth.

"The five atmospheric influences enter the nostrils and are stored by the heart and the lungs and then they are allowed to rise. The five colors restore brightness and light. The (musical) sounds are manifestations of talent and ability. The five flavors enter the

10. The part of the sentence in brackets was added by Wang Ping.
11. 靈 神 Ling Shên, a god who answers his worshippers (Mathews).
12. The five colors: red, green, yellow, white, black.
13. The five flavors: bitter, sour, sweet, pungent, salt.

mouth and are stored by the stomach. The flavors which are stored nourish the five atmospheric influences, and when these influences are well-blended they produce saliva. Together all these influences help to perfect the mind, which then begins to function spontaneously."

The Emperor asked: "How can you explain the outer appearances (象) of the viscera?"

Ch'i Po answered: "The heart is the root of life and causes the versatility of the spiritual faculties. The heart influences the face and fills the pulse with blood. Within Yang, the principle of light and life, the heart acts as the Great Yang which permeates the climate of Summer.

"The lungs are the origin of breath and the dwelling of the animal spirits or inferior soul. The lungs influence the body hair and have their effect upon the skin. Within Yang, the lungs act as the great Yin which permeates the climate in Fall.

"The kidneys (testicles) call to life that which is dormant and sealed up; they are the natural organ for storing away, and they are the place where the secretions are lodged. The kidneys influence the hair on the head and have an effect upon the bones. Within Yin the kidneys act as the lesser Yin which permeates the climate of Winter.

"The liver causes utmost weariness and is the dwelling place of the soul, or spiritual part of man that ascends to Heaven. The liver influences the nails and is effective upon the muscles; it brings forth animal desires and vigor. The taste connected with the liver is sour and the color connected with the liver is green. Within Yang the liver acts as the lesser Yang which permeates the air in Spring.

"In the stomach, the lower intestines, the small intestines, the three foci, the groin and the bladder, one can find the basic principle for the public granaries and the encampment of a regiment. These organs are called 'vessels', and have the power of transforming the dregs and the sediment, and cause the flavors to revolve so that they enter the vessels and leave them. These organs influence the lips and cause the flesh around them to be of light color; these organs are effective upon the flesh and the muscles. The flavor connected with these organs is sweet and the color is yellow. They belong to the organs of Yin which permeates the climate of the earth.

"In general one can say that the eleven viscera either receive from the gall bladder or expel into it.

"When people have one pulse full and abundant, the disease is in the region of the lesser Yang. When two pulses are full and abundant, the disease is in the region of the Great Yang; when three pulses are full and abundant, the disease is located in the region of the 'sunlight'. When four pulses are full and abundant, the disease has come to an end and the powers above act as regulators of Yang.

"When the 'inch' (寸) pulse at the wrist beats once fully and abundantly, the disease is located in the region of the absolute Yin. When the 'inch' pulse at the wrist beats twice fully and abundantly, the disease is located in the region of the lesser Yin. When the 'inch' pulse at the wrist beats three times fully and abundantly, the disease is located in the region of the Great Yin. When the 'inch' pulse beats four times fully and abundantly, the disease has come to an end and the powers above close Yin.

"When all the 'inch' pulses at the wrist are concurrent and flourishing, the four pulses join and come to an end, and the powers above intermittently close and regulate the pulse. Through this system of closing and regulating the pulse there can never be a surplus. When the essence of Heaven and Earth has come to an end (has been exhausted), death follows."[14]

14. Wang Ping explains: the absolute Yin is the region of the liver; the lesser Yin is the region of the kidneys; and the great Yin is the region of the stomach.

10. *Treatise on the Five Viscera in Relation to Their Part in Perfecting Life*

The heart is in accord with the pulse. The complexion of a person shows when the heart is in a splendid condition. The heart rules over the kidneys.

The lungs are connected with the skin. The condition of the body hair shows when the lungs are in a splendid and flourishing condition. The lungs rule over the heart.

The liver is connected (in accord) with the muscles. The condition of the finger and toe nails shows when the liver is in a splendid and flourishing condition. The liver rules over the lungs.

The spleen is connected with the flesh. The color and appearance of the lips show when the stomach is in a splendid and flourishing condition. The liver rules over the lungs.

The kidneys are connected with the bones. The condition of the hair on the head shows when the lungs are in a splendid and flourishing condition. The kidneys rule over the spleen.

Hence if too much salt is used in food, the pulse hardens, tears make their appearance and the complexion changes. If too much bitter flavor is used in food, the skin becomes withered and the body hair falls out. If too much pungent flavor is used in food, the muscles become knotty and the finger and toe nails wither and decay. If too much sour flavor is used in food, the flesh hardens and wrinkles and the lips become slack. If too much sweet flavor is used in food, the bones ache and the hair on the head falls out. These then are the injuries which can be brought about by the five flavors.

We know that the heart craves the bitter flavor; the lungs crave the pungent flavor; the liver craves the sour flavor; the spleen craves the sweet flavor; and the kidneys crave the salty flavor. These are the correct combinations of the five flavors, and the state of the viscera can be observed by the appearance and color (of their related external organs).

When their color is green like grass they are without life; when their color is yellow like that of oranges they are without life; when their color is black like coal they are without life; when their color is red like blood they are without life; when their color is white like dried and withered bones they are without life. This is how the five colors manifest death.

When the viscera are green like the kingfisher's wings they are full of life; when they are red like a cock's comb they are full of life; when they are yellow like the belly of a crab they are full of life; when they are white like the grease of pigs they are full of life; and when they are black like the wings of a crow they are full of life. This is how the five colors manifest life.

The color of life displayed by the heart is like the vermilion red lining of a white silk robe; the color of life displayed by the lungs is like the lucky red lining of a white silk robe; the color of life displayed by the liver is like the violet lining of a white silk robe; the color of life displayed by the stomach is like the juniper berry colored lining of a white silk robe; the color of life displayed by the kidneys is like the purple lining of a white silk robe. These are the colorful and magnificent external signs of life of the five viscera.

Each color and flavor belongs to one of the five viscera: white belongs to the lungs just like the pungent flavor; red belongs to the heart just like the bitter flavor; green belongs to the liver just like the sour flavor; yellow belongs to the stomach just like the sweet flavor; black belongs to the kidneys just like the salty flavor.

Thus white also belongs to the skin; red belongs to the pulse; green belongs to the muscles; yellow belongs to the flesh; and black belongs to the bones.

The pulse is connected with the eyes; the marrow is connected with the brain; the muscles are connected with the joints; the blood is connected with the heart; and the breath is connected with the lungs.

The four limbs and their eight flexible joints[1] are in use from early morning until late at night. When people lie down to rest the blood flows back to the liver. When the liver receives the blood it strengthens the vision.[2] When the feet receive blood it strengthens the footsteps. When the palm of the hand receives blood the hand can be used to grasp. When the fingers receive blood they can be used to carry.

When a person is exposed to the wind, either lying down to rest or walking about, his blood will be affected. The blood then coagulates within the flesh, and the result is numbness in the hands and the feet;[3] when it coagulates within the pulse the blood ceases to circulate beneficially;[4] when the blood coagulates within the feet it causes pains and chills.[5]

When the blood goes into these three organs [flesh, pulse, and feet] and cannot turn back, its passage becomes empty and numbness and disagreeableness follow.

Man has twelve groups of large ducts or main vessels[6] and three

1. Wang Ping explains the flexible joints as elbows, knees, wrists, and ankles.
2. Wang Ping explains: "The eyes are connected with the liver, therefore they are strengthened when the liver receives blood."
3. Wang Ping explains 痺 to mean 瘀痺.
4. Wang Ping explains: 泣 to mean 血行不利.
5. Wang Ping explains 厥 to mean 足逆冷.
6. Wang Ping explains: the places where the main arteries meet are called 'great caves' (大谷), or great ducts.

hundred and sixty-four small ducts or '*loh* vessels' (絡),[7] and twelve vessels of lesser importance. They all protect the life-giving element and prevent evil influences from entering. When acupuncture is applied it causes evil influences to depart.

At the beginning of an examination for disease one must investigate whether the pulses of the five viscera are interrupted and one must control them. In order to know (the proper time) for this beginning one must first establish which of the ten stems is to be the first month of the year.

The five indications that the functions of the five viscera are interrupted are the five pulses. Headaches and madness are indicated by the lower pulse being empty and slow and the upper pulse being quick and full. When these diseases are examined at the pulse of the foot, it is felt that they are in the region of the lesser Yin and the Great Yang, which indicates that they have also entered the kidneys.

Lack of discernment causes evil. Obscured eyesight and impaired hearing are indicated by the lower pulse being full and the upper pulse being empty. When these diseases are examined at the pulse of the foot, one feels that they are in the region of the lesser Yang and the Great Yang; this indicates that the disease has entered the liver.

When the stomach is too full, dropsical swellings of the limbs, the diaphragm, the ribs and the flanks occur; then the pulse is rebellious below and flourishing above. If these diseases are examined at the pulse of the foot, one feels that they are in the region of the 'sunlight' and the Great Yang.

When there are pains at the heart and headaches the disease is located within the thorax. When these diseases are examined at the pulse of the hands, one feels that they are in the region of the Great Yang and the lesser Yin.

Thus it can be pointed out and distinguished whether the pulses are small or large, slippery (滑) or rough (澀), light (浮) or heavy (沈). The external appearances of the five viscera can be put in the same categories.

The five viscera are connected with the five musical notes, which can be discerned and recognized. The five colors can be used for subtle examinations and help the eyes in the examination of diseases,

---

7. The places where the *loh* vessels (絡) meet are called 'small caves' (小 谿), or small ducts. (See Wong and Wu, p. 19.)

and if one has the ability of combining the significance of the pulses with the significance of the colors a complete diagnosis can be made.

When the pulse has a red appearance and there is an obstinate cough, the examiner says that there is amassed air within (the heart) and it is dangerous to eat at this particular time. The disease is known as 'numbness (痹) of the heart.' It is contracted through external evil influences, causing anxiety and emptying the heart while the evil influences follow into it.

When the pulse has a white appearance and there is a light cough, and the pulse is empty above and full below, the examiner can suspect that there is amassed air within the thorax, causing shortness of breath and a hollow sound. The name of the disease is 'numbness of the lungs' and the external evidences are chills and fevers. This disease is caused through toxicity which influences the inner body.

When the pulse has a green appearance and the pulses at the left and the right hand are pressed down for a long time, the examiner will find that there is air amassed within the heart which descends into the limbs and flanks. The name of the disease is 'numbness of the liver.' This disease is contracted through chills and dampness and is associated with ruptures (疝) affecting the loins; then the feet hurt and the head aches.

When the pulse has a yellow appearance, the pulse becomes large and slow and there is amassed air in the spleen. The examiner will find that there is troublesome gas. The disease is known as 'rupture caused by troublesome gas.' Women too are victims of this disease, which can be contracted through perspiration upon the four limbs when exposed to wind (當 風).

When the pulse has a black appearance the upper pulse is strong and big, and the examiner will find that there is amassed air in the small intestines, which is the region of Yin. The name of the disease is 'numbness of the kidneys.' This illness can be cured by bathing in pure water and lying down to rest.

Every disease has a symbol through the variety of the five colors of the pulse. When the surface is yellow and the eyes see green, when the surface is yellow and the eyes see red, when the surface is yellow and the eyes see white, when the surface is yellow and the eyes see black, death will not strike.[8] But when the surface is green and the eyes see red, when the surface is red and the eyes see white,

8. Yellow is the color of the stomach.

when the surface is green and the eyes see black, when the surface is black and the eyes see white, and when the surface is red and the eyes see green, death will strike.[9]

9. Wang Ping explains: If the surface (complexion) is yellow then it is an indication that the stomach is full of life-giving spirit and health; if the complexion is not yellow there will be death because of lack of vital essence emanating from the stomach; the stomach is the most essential of the five viscera.

11. *Treatise on the Method of Distinguishing the Five Viscera*

The Yellow Emperor asked: "I understand that scholars versed in prescriptions are uncertain whether the brain and the marrow govern the viscera, or whether it is the stomach that governs the viscera, or whether the viscera govern the six bowels.

"May I inquire whether the natural tendency of these organs is to assist each other or to oppose each other? Tell me, for I do not know their principles and ways. I am eager to hear your explanation."

Ch'i Po answered: "The brain, the marrow, the bones, the pulse, the gall, and the womb of the woman, these six organs, have been produced by the atmosphere of the earth. They all are viscera belonging to Yin and they are the natural symbols of the earth; therefore they store and do not dispel, and their name is 'unfailing and preserving intestines.'

"The stomach, the lower intestines, the small intestines, the three foci, and the bladder, these five viscera, have an evil odor and their name is 'conducting and transforming intestines.' Within these nothing can remain for a long time, for they transport and dispel.

"The rectum too is part of the five viscera and prevents the water and the grain from being retained too long within the viscera.

"The so-called five viscera store up the essences of life and do not dispel them: since they must be filled they cannot be solid.

"The six bowels conduct and transform substance and do not store, therefore they are solid and cannot be filled.

"Hence water and grain enter the mouth and pass into the stomach, which becomes full while the bowels are still hollow. When the food (water and grain) descends, then the bowels become full and the stomach becomes again empty. Thus one can say: when the bowels and viscera are solid they cannot be filled, and when they must be filled they cannot be solid."

The Emperor asked: "Is the 'inch' (寸) pulse at the wrist[1] alone indicative for the five viscera?"

Ch'i Po answered: "The stomach acts as a place of accumulation for water and grain and as a source of supply for the six bowels.

"The five flavors enter the mouth and are stored by the stomach in order to bring nourishment to the five viscera and to the breath of life. The five viscera are connected with the 'inch' pulse which is active in the region of the great Yin.

"Thus all force of life and all the flavors go towards the stomach, where they are digested and then become apparent in the 'inch' pulse at the wrist.

"The five atmospheric influences enter the nostrils and are stored in the heart and in the lungs. When heart and lungs are sick then the nose cannot function properly. In order to cure these diseases one must examine whether they extend farther down, the pulse must be watched and its scope and tendencies must be observed.

"Those who would restrain the demons and the gods (good and evil spirits) cannot attain virtue by speaking about it; and those who dislike acupuncture cannot achieve ingenious results by speaking about them.

"Those who do not allow treatment of a disease will certainly not be cured, and treatment by force never has good results."

---

1. Wang Ping explains 氣 口 to mean 寸 口 .

Book 4

12. *The Different Methods of Treatment and the Appropriate Prescriptions*

THE Yellow Emperor asked: "When the physicians treat diseases, do they treat each disease differently from the others and can they all be healed?"

Ch'i Po answered: "Yes, they can all be healed according to the physical features of the place where one lives.

"Beginning and creation come from the East. Fish and salt are the products of water and ocean and of the shores near the water. The people of the regions of the East eat fish and crave salt; their living is tranquil and their food delicious. Fish causes people to burn within (thirst), and the eating of salt injures (defeats) the blood. Therefore the people of these regions are all of dark complexion and careless and lax in their principles. Their diseases are ulcers, which are most properly treated with acupuncture by means of a needle of flint. Thus the treatment with acupuncture with a needle of flint has its origin in the regions of the East.

"Precious metals and jade come from the regions of the West. The dwellings in the West are built of pebbles and sandstone. Nature (Heaven and Earth) exerts itself to bring a good harvest. The people of these regions live on hills and, because of the great amount of wind, water, and soil, become robust and energetic. The people of these regions wear no clothes other than those of coarse woolen stuff or coarse matting. They eat good and variegated food and therefore they are flourishing and fertile. Hence evil cannot injure their external bodies, and if they get diseases they strike at the inner body. These diseases are most successfully cured with poison medicines. Thus the treatment with poison medicines comes from the West.

"The North is the region of storing and laying by. The country is hilly and mountainous, there are biting cold winds, frost and ice. The people of these regions find pleasure in living in this wilderness, and they live on milk products. The extreme cold causes many diseases. These diseases are most fittingly treated with cauterization by burning the dried tinder of the artemisia (moxa). Hence the treatment with cauterization has its origin in the regions of the North.

"Nourishment and growth come from the South. The Sun makes the life of those who live in the regions of the South plentiful and nourishing. Although there is water beneath the earth, the soil is deficient, (but) it collects dew and mist. The people who live in the regions of the South crave sour food and curd. They are secretive and soft in their ways and attached to the red color. Their diseases are bent and contracted muscles and numbness. These diseases are most fittingly treated with acupuncture with fine needles. Hence the treatment with the nine needles comes from the South.

"The region of the center, the Earth, is level and moist. Everything that is created by the Universe meets in the center and is absorbed by the Earth. The people of the regions of the center eat mixed food and do not (suffer or weary at their) toil. Their diseases are many: they suffer from complete paralysis and chills and fever. These diseases are most fittingly treated with breathing exercises, massage of skin and flesh, and exercises of hands and feet. Hence the treatment with breathing exercises, massage and exercises of the limbs has its origin in the center regions.

"The ancient sages combined these various treatments for the purpose of cure, and each patient received the treatment that was most fitting for him. These treatments were so extraordinary and so different in each case that all diseases were healed. Thus the circumstances and needs of each disease were ascertained and the principle of the art of healing became known."

13. *Treatise on the Transmittal of the Essence and the Transformation of the Life-giving Principle*

The Yellow Emperor asked: "I understand that in olden times the treatment of diseases consisted merely of the transmittal of the Essence and the transformation of the life-giving principle. One could invoke the gods and this was the way to treat. The present generation treats internal diseases with the (5) poison medicines and they treat external diseases with acupuncture, and sometimes the patients are healed and sometimes the patients are not healed.   How can you explain this?"

Ch'i Po answered:"In former times man lived among birds, beasts and reptiles; he worked, moved and stirred in order to avoid and to escape the cold and the darkness, and he sought a dwelling into which he could flee from the heat.   Within him there were no family ties which bound him with love; on the outside there were no officials who could guide out and correct his physical appearance.   Into this tranquil and peaceful era evil influences could not penetrate deeply. Therefore poison medicines were not needed for the treatment of internal diseases, and acupuncture was not needed for the cure of external diseases.   Hence it was sufficient to transmit the Essence and to invoke the gods; and this was the way to treat.

"But the present world is a different one.   Grief, calamity, and evil cause inner bitterness, while the body receives wounds from the outside; moreover there is neglect against the laws of the four seasons, there is disobedience and rebellion and there are those who violate the customs of what is proper during the cold of Winter and the heat of Summer.   Reprimands are in vain.   Evil influences strike from early morning until late at night; they injure the five viscera, the bones and the marrow within the body, and externally they injure the mind and reduce its intelligence and they also injure the muscles and the flesh.   Hence the minor illnesses are bound to become grave and the serious diseases are bound to result in death. Therefore the invocation of the gods is no longer the way to cure."

The Emperor said: "Very good!   I should like to be near a sick person and to observe when death strikes.   The sudden end of life fills me with curiosity and doubts.   I wish to know whether the point of death can be as clearly ascertained as the light of the sun and the moon."

Ch'i Po answered: "The ancient emperors held the complexion and the pulse in great honor.   The early scholars proclaimed the doctrine of these indications.   In ancient times the scholar borrowed from and relied upon the system of the four seasons; he relied upon the complexion and the pulse and understood their meaning.

"The sages combined water, fire, wood, metal, and earth, the four seasons and the eight winds, the four cardinal points, the Zenith and the Nadir (六 合), and they held them as inseparable and constant. They underwent changes and transformations by mutually influencing each other, and one could observe their wonderful and subtle power and one would know their needs. Thus if one wants to find the meaning of these above-mentioned forces one will find them expressed in the complexion and the pulse.

"The complexion corresponds with the sun; the pulse corresponds with the moon. If one is constant in one's search for their meaning one will discover the importance of the complexion and the pulse. But the complexion undergoes a change according to the respective pulse of the four seasons, and this change was held in high esteem by the old emperors; there they agreed with the sages, and thus death was relegated to the far distance, whereas life was brought close.

"When the medieval scholars treated diseases they used hot water and liquid treatment for ten days in order to remove the five illnesses of numbness,[1] which are brought about by the eight winds. When this ten-day treatment did not terminate the disease, they prescribed thyme and the roots of herbs. And when the stalks and roots did not show any alleviating effect, the topmost branches and the farthest roots, swallowed as medicine, were considered effective in the termination of the evil influences.[2]

"The treatment in this past age was quite different. It was not based upon the four seasons, there was no knowledge of sun and moon, there was no examination as to obedience or disobedience (towards the laws of nature). In order to terminate physical illnesses and to bring health, external diseases were treated with acupuncture and internal diseases with hot water or soups, and liquid medicines.

"Poor medical workmanship is neglectful and careless and must therefore be combatted, because a disease that is not completely cured can easily breed new disease or there can be a relapse of the old disease."

The Emperor said: "I should like to be informed about the essential doctrines (of healing)."

Ch'i Po answered: "The most important requirement of the art of healing is that no mistakes or neglect occur. There should be no doubt or confusion as to the application of the meaning of complexion and pulse. These are the maxims of the art of healing. When those

1. Wang Ping explains 五 痹, the five illnesses of numbness, are those of the skin, the flesh, the muscles, the bones, and the pulse.
2. Wang Ping adds that these roots and branches should be simmered or fried in oil.

who rebelled against the laws of nature obtained power, the medicines prepared from the topmost branches and roots were no longer given, the divine spirit perished and the country deteriorated. But as soon as the rebels were removed all good practices were revived by the succeeding Spiritual Men who had attained Tao, the right way of life."

The Emperor said: "I understand the importance and the need for teachers, teachers who can proclaim the theory that one cannot separate the complexion from the pulse—the doctrine which I consider pure wisdom."

Ch'i Po answered: "The utmost in the art of healing can be achieved when there is unity."

The Emperor inquired: "What is meant by unity?"

Ch'i Po answered: "When the minds of the people are closed and wisdom is locked out they remain tied to disease. Yet their feelings and desires should be investigated and made known, their wishes and ideas should be followed; and then it becomes apparent that those who have attained spirit and energy are flourishing and prosperous, while those perish who lose their spirit and energy."

The Emperor exclaimed: "Excellent, indeed!"

14. *Treatise on the Treatment with Hot Water, Liquid Medicines, the Lees of Wine, and Sweet Wine*

The Yellow Emperor asked: "How can one prepare soups and clear liquids and even lees of wine and sweet wine from the five kinds of grain?"[1]

Ch'i Po replied: "One must use paddy rice and steam it. The stalks of the paddy rice serve as firewood. When the steaming of the rice is completed, the rice (extract) is strong."

The Emperor inquired: "How is this possible?"

Ch'i Po answered: "The effect is obtained by mixing the products of Heaven and Earth, the exalted and the base substances, in proper proportion. Hence if this can be done and the plants be cut at the proper season, the potion will be strong."

The Emperor said: "In ancient times, although the sages prescribed soups and hot water, the lees of wine and sweet wine as

1. The five grains are: glutinous millet, wheat, millet, rice, and beans.

medicines, they did not know how to use them.   Is this the case?"

Ch'i Po answered: "From olden times the sages prescribed soups, liquids, the lees of wine and sweet wine and medicines, but their special emphasis was on the preparation.   Thus from olden times these soups and liquid medicines were prepared but not swallowed as medicines.

"In medieval times, when morality deteriorated, these medicines were first taken at the time when evil influences appeared and they worked very effectively."

The Emperor said: "The present generation should not be like the medieval world."

Ch'i Po said: "The present generation must respect (齊) the poisonous medicines, which assault the diseases within their bodies, and they should hold in awe acupuncture and treatment with moxa, which cure the diseases of the external body."

The Emperor asked: "When the body is worn out and the blood is exhausted, is it still possible to achieve good results?"

Ch'i Po replied: "No, because there is no more energy left."

The Emperor inquired: "What does it mean, there is no more energy left?"

Ch'i Po answered: "This is the way of acupuncture: if man's vitality and energy do not propel his own will his disease cannot be cured.

"Nowadays vitality and energy are considered the foundation of life; in order to keep them flourishing they must be protected and the life-giving force must rule.   When this force does not support life, its foundation will dissolve, and how can a disease be cured when there is no spiritual energy within the body?"

The Emperor said: "Thus life itself is really the beginning of illness!   Minute particles first enter the body through the skin, and all physicians of skilful workmanship, those who are renowned, call this group 'stubborn diseases' (逆).   If they cannot be cured by means of acupuncture, not even good medicine can bring a cure. Nowadays the good physicians all have developed a definite method: they guard the fate of the parents, of kin, of brother, of strangers and of close friends.   They perceive the sounds and noises of the day with their ears and they observe the colors of the day with their eyes; and how could they relax before the illness has improved?"

Ch'i Po replied: "Illness is comparable to the root; good medical work is comparable to the topmost branch or a beacon. If this root is not reached, the evil influences cannot be subjugated. This is what I want to say."

The Emperor said: "Those who are not obedient to the smallest fraction can yet live; but Yang, the principle of life within their five viscera, is exhausted. Saliva and liquid secretions act as rim for their animal (or inferior) soul, which dwells in isolation. The spirit is confined to the interior of the body, while wasteful and destructive airs attack from the outside. The body can no longer wear clothes and protect its four extremities. Thus distress can move into the lungs (center), and the entry of life-giving force is impeded from within while the body is neglected at the outside. How can a cure be effected under these conditions?"

Ch'i Po answered: "The fairest treatment is to weigh and to consider carefully removal, as well as cutting and scooping out exposed and spoiled particles. Even if they are ulcerated one should move the four extremities slowly and clothe them warmly. One should criticize and correct the faults in the patients' mode of life; one should restore their bodies and open the anus so that the bowels can be cleansed, and so that the secretions come at the proper time and serve the five viscera which belong to Yang, the principle of life.

"One should put in order the five viscera which were remiss and cleanse and purify them. Then the secretions are certain to produce life, and the body contains flourishing bones and flesh without further help; they all help and protect each other, and thus the life-giving force becomes strong and peaceful."

The Emperor said: "Wonderful indeed!"

15. *Treatise on the Precious Plans*

The Yellow Emperor said: "I understand that you take into consideration that strange and rare occurrences and those which are constant and regular have different indications and cannot be treated alike."

Ch'i Po answered: "I take into consideration the degree of the disease, and whether it is light or grave, rare or frequent. When I speak about rare diseases I use the utmost effort in following Tao (the Right Way). I discriminate between the five colors and the changes of the pulse and take into consideration whether they are rare or ordinary. I follow Tao in both cases.

"Once the spirit has turned away it will—as a rule—not return. If, however, it should return, it will not improve; thus the moving power of nature is lost. The importance of the calculations of the colors and the pulse is great, although those calculations must be done subtly. These calculations are written down on precious tablets which are said to contain precious secrets.[1]

"The patient's appearance (color) must be watched high and low, left and right—each where it is most essential. When the complexion is light the patient should be treated with soups and liquid medicines for ten days, and then the disease should disappear. When the complexion is dark the patient must be treated in the same manner for twenty-one days. When the complexion is very dark the patient must be given lees of wine and fermented liquor for one hundred days. When the complexion of the face is young and fresh (and yet the patient does not improve), the treatment should not exceed one hundred days. When the pulse is deficient and tense and the breath interrupted death will occur. When there is a revival of the illness and the pulse becomes slow and vacant death will ensue.

"The appearance and complexion must be watched high and low, to the left and to the right, for each has its significance. When the color rises it indicates rebellion; when it recedes it indicates submission.

"Woman's right pulse indicates disorder, her left pulse indicates order; man's left pulse indicates disorder, while his right pulse indicates order.[2]

"When serious changes occur in Yang, death ensues, and when they occur in Yin death also ensues, because then Yin and Yang oppose each other. For in regard to medical treatment one must also take into consideration that the two forces in nature can attack each other on unusual occasions and even at regular occurrences. Thus every undertaking must be prefigured.

1. 著 之 玉 版 命 曰 合 玉 機.
2. Wang Pang explains: Left represents Yang, the male principle, therefore man's left pulse indicates disorder. Right represents Yin, the female principle, therefore woman's right pulse indicates disorder.

"When the pulse is seized hastily numbness and lameness ensue, followed by a variation of fevers and chills. When the pulse is isolated it will exhaust the breath, and when the breath is exhausted and empty it will strike at the blood. Isolation is comparable to disorder, while slowness is comparable to order.

"When one follows the right method for the treatment of rare and frequent diseases, one bases it upon the great Yin. If by doing so one cannot overcome the disease it is called 'stubborn,' and when it is stubborn death will ensue. If by following these methods one overcomes the disease it is called 'obedient,' and when it is obedient the patient becomes again lively and active.

"When the eight winds and the four seasons overcome death they restore the body to its original state; but those who are disobedient to the laws of nature are not restored to their original state.

"This is the end of this treatise."

16. *Treatise on the Important Examination of the Invariable Rules of Death*

The Yellow Emperor asked: "I desire to examine (the rules of death). What can you tell me?"

Ch'i Po answered: "In the first and the second month the heavenly breath created the earth, the breath of the earth created man, and the breath animated his liver. In the third and fourth month the heavenly climate firmly established the earth, and the climate of the earth brought forth a definite form for man, and the breath animated his spleen. In the fifth and sixth month the heavenly climate flourished and the climate of the earth elevated man, and the breath animated his head. In the seventh and eighth month Yin, the female element of darkness and death, began to kill man, while the breath animated his lungs. In the ninth and tenth month Yin began to consolidate, and the subtle influence that animates the earth began to obstruct the breath of man, which had now reached his heart. In the eleventh and twelfth month frost again congealed the earth, whose breath unites with the breath of man in animating his kidneys.

"But Spring pierces and scatters the frost and disperses and breaks the ice. It also stimulates the flow of blood and its interruptions.

The blood is then induced to flow in the intervals of respiration, thus creating circulation.

"Summer penetrates the blood-vessels (絡) so that the blood becomes exhausted and ceases to circulate. And since the circulation of the air is also obstructed, there is extreme pain, and diseases are brought about which must be expelled.

"Autumn penetrates the skin, and this is in accord with the principles of nature; the upper and the lower pulses work alike, the energy undergoes a transformation and ceases to function.

"Winter penetrates the mind and shatters reason and intelligence. That which was firmly built is now undermined and the mind is scattered.

"Spring, Summer, Fall, Winter, each of the seasons has a special effect, and together they have a method. When Spring has a stimulating effect, Summer has a distributing effect. It disturbs breathing and causes licentiousness and immorality which, in turn, cause diseases of the bones and the marrow, which cannot be cured. Because of this man cannot enjoy his food and consequently his energy is reduced.

"When Spring has a stimulating effect, Autumn has a scattering effect; it makes the muscles bent and crooked, and the rebellious forces form a ring, thus inducing a cough which cannot be improved; it frightens and alarms people at special times and makes them cry.

"When Spring has a stimulating effect, Winter distributes the evil influences which become manifest within the viscera, and causes dropsical swellings, which cannot be cured. Moreover the people are given to jabbering talk.

"When Summer has a stimulating effect, Spring distributes diseases which cannot be cured, and thus people become idolent.

"When Summer has a stimulating effect, Autumn distributes diseases which cannot be cured, and thus people feel within their hearts the desire not to talk of their worries and troubles; they act like people about to be apprehended and seized.

"When Summer has a stimulating effect, Winter distributes diseases which cannot be cured; they reduce the vitality of the people, although the people are apt to be violent and enraged.

"When Fall has a stimulating effect, Spring distributes diseases which cannot be cured and this causes alarm. The people are filled with the desire to neglect and forget that which they have just begun.

"When Fall has a stimulating effect, Summer distributes diseases which cannot be cured, and this increases the people's desire to lie down to rest and to get peaceful sleep (瘻 = 寢).

"When Fall has a stimulating effect, Winter distributes diseases which cannot be cured, causing people to have a desire for lying down to sleep; but although they sleep they are conscious.

"When Winter has a stimulating effect, Fall distributes diseases which cannot be cured, causing people to be very thirsty.

"In general all stimulation affects the chest, the mind, and the stomach, and it is necessary to avoid that they (in turn) affect the five viscera. Once the stimulation has penetrated into the heart, the heart becomes encircled and death ensues. When the stimulation penetrates into the spleen death ensues within five days; when it penetrates into the diaphragm (鬲 - 膈) all inner organs receive injuries, their resulting diseases are difficult to cure and within a period not exceeding one year those afflicted will most certainly die.

"When one has been successful in protecting the five viscera from being penetrated, one knows whether the diseases are stubborn or curable. The curable ones are located in the diaphragm and in the spleen and the kidneys; but when this is not known the disease will recur.

"When the thorax and the belly are penetrated it is necessary to give immediate attention to these organs, because, when this penetration is known, it can be arrested and cured and the penetration can be isolated above.

"When acupuncture does not cure it must be repeated. The needle for acupuncture must be applied quietly and with utmost care. When acupuncture is applied for swellings the needle must be shaken. When acupuncture is applied for diseases affecting the blood vessels, the needle should not be shaken. This is the way to apply acupuncture."

The Emperor said: "I desire to be informed about death in relation to the twelve blood vessels."

Ch'i Po answered: "When the pulse of the great Yang causes the end, the pupil of the eye cannot revolve and it is turned upwards but in the wrong direction, and convulsions occur; the color of the eyes is white. Life is interrupted, sweat appears and when it is all spent death follows.

"When the lesser Yang causes the end, the ears turn deaf, the hundred joints all relax completely, the eyes are encircled and cease to function, all connections within the body break up and within a day and a half the patient is almost dead. At first his complexion turns green, later it turns white and then death follows.

"When [the region of] the 'sunlight' causes the end, mouth and eyes move very well, but then the patient gets frightened and begins to talk wildly and incoherently. His color turns yellow, and his arteries above and below are full and without sensation; then the end follows.

"When the lesser Yin causes the end, the face turns black, the teeth protrude and turn foul, the belly swells and closes up, and circulation above and below ceases; and then the end follows.

"When the great Yin causes the end, the belly swells and becomes closed; the patient cannot breathe, and then belching and vomiting occur. Belching is the indication of contrary air and in this case the face is red. When breathing is impossible movement above and below ceases, and the face turns black; skin and body hair feel dry and burnt and the end follows.

"When the 'absolute' Yin causes the end, there is heat within the throat and the patient is given over to severe heart trouble; the tongue curls up and becomes spongy and porous and shrinks towards the upper gum; and then the end follows.

"This is the story of death in relation to the twelve main vessels."

Book 5

17. Treatise on the Importance of the Pulse and the Subtle Skill of its Examination

THE Yellow Emperor asked: "What is the way of medical treatment?"

Ch'i Po answered: "The way of medical treatment is to be consistent. It should be executed at dawn when the breath of Yin [the female principle in nature] has not yet begun to stir and when the breath of Yang [the male principle of life and light] has not yet begun to diffuse, when food and drink have not yet been taken, when the twelve main vessels (經 脉) are not yet abundant and when the *lo* vessels (絡 脉) are stirred up thoroughly; when vigor and energy are not yet disturbed—at that particular time one should examine what has happened to the pulse.

"One should feel whether the pulse is in motion or whether it is still and one should observe attentively and with skill. One should examine the five colors and the five viscera, whether they suffer from excess or whether they show an insufficiency, and one should examine the six bowels whether they are strong or weak. One should investigate the appearance of the body whether it is flourishing or deteriorating. One should use all these five examinations and combine their results, and then one will be able to decide upon the share of life and death.

"The pulse is the store-house of the blood. When the pulse beats are long and the strokes markedly prolonged (長), then the constitution of the pulse is well regulated; when the pulse beats are short and without volume (短), then the constitution of the pulse is out of order. When the pulse is quick, and contains six beats to one cycle of respiration (數), then it indicates heart trouble; and when the pulse is large (大) the disease becomes grave.

"When the upper pulse is abundant then its impulse is strong; when the lower pulse is abundant then it indicates flatulence. When the pulse is irregular and tremulous and the beats occur at irregular intervals (代), then the impulse of life fades; when the pulse is slender [smaller than feeble, but still perceptible, thin like a silk thread] (細), then the impulse of life is small. When the pulse is small and fine, slow and short like scraping bamboo with a knife (濇), then it indicates that the heart is irritated and painful.

"When the force of the pulse is turbid and the color disturbed like a bubbling well, it is a sign that disease has entered the body, the color has become corrupted and the constitution delicate. And when the constitution is delicate it will be broken up like the strings of a lute and die. Therefore, it is desirable to understand the force of the five viscera.

"Red tends to serve as white lining, but vermillion red does not incline to change into ochre; white wants to be like the feathers of a goose and not like the color of salt. Green wants to be like the blue of the heavens, but the glossy and shining surface of jade does not want to be indigo blue. Yellow wants to be like the bindings of a net, put out to catch a cock-bird, but yellow does not want to be like loess. Black wants to be like a thick layer, but the black color of the varnish-tree does not want to be like the grayish-green of the earth. Much can be deduced from the subtle and delicate phenomena of the five colors, and [when they act as mentioned above] the life of the patient will not be a long one.[1]

"But those who are skilful and clever in examination observe every living creature. They distinguish black and white; they examine whether the pulse is short or long. When they mistake a long pulse for a short one and when they mistake white for black or commit similar errors, then it is a sign that their skill has deteriorated.

"The five viscera which are within the body must be guarded. When the viscera within are flourishing they are full of life-giving force and are able to overcome injury and fear, and the tones emitted are harmonious and similar to those which come from within a family mansion; this means that the air within the body is humid, or as if one said that the tones are fine and delicate and that noise has been terminated and made unable to continue; and all this means that the life-giving force has supremacy over the disease.

"When the clothes which are worn by a person are not well arranged it means, according to a proverb: Good and evil cannot be

1. Wang Ping explains: When the ochre color, the color of the salt, indigo blue, and the gray color can be seen, it means the ruin of all appearance and therefore life will not be long.

hidden, be they near or far away; it is thus provided by the gods. And when granaries and store-houses do not store provisions, it is as though doors and gateways had no meaning and importance.[2]

"When water and wells do not cease to run it is as if the bladder were not able to retain liquid. Those who pay heed to these functions will live and those who neglect to attend to these functions will die, for the five viscera are the stronghold of the body.

"The head is the home of skill and intelligence. When man keeps the head bowed he sees only what is deep below and his vitality and spirit will be broken.

"The back is the home of the structure of the thorax. When the back is bent as a consequence of carrying heavy burdens, the thorax will be ruined.

"The middle of the loins is the home of the kidneys; when they do not have the power to transmit and to change, the kidneys will be exhausted.

"The knees are the home of the muscles. When the muscles have no elasticity and cannot rise and bend at will, a hunchback will develop and the muscles will deteriorate.

"The bones are the home of the marrow. When for a long time one has not been able to stand up and to walk, then one flaps and shakes and the bones will deteriorate.

"When strength is preserved then life is safe; when one neglects to preserve strength then it means death."

Ch'i Po went on to say:[3] "Those who act contrary to the laws of the four seasons and live in excess have insufficient secretions and dissipate in their duties. When they go beyond the mark in the fulfilment of their duties or when they perform their duties incompletely, their secretions are small. When their performance of their duties is incomplete, they live in excess and this causes dissipation. And since under these conditions Yin and Yang do not correspond to each other, a disease results which is known to influence the center (bar) pulse (關)."

The Emperor asked: "Is not the pulse influenced by the four seasons? How can one know where the disease is located? How can one know the changes a disease may undergo? How can one

2. Wang Ping explains: Granaries are equal to the stomach and the gates are equal to the anus.
3. Wang Ping adds: "although there was no preceding question."

know whether a disease is at first located in the interior? How can one know whether it may not at first be located at the outside? I beg you to answer these five questions."

Ch'i Po answered: "Please bear in mind that the power of Heaven is great and that it can change ill luck for the better. Outside of all living creation and within the Universe are transformations brought about by Heaven and Earth and by the interrelation of Yin and Yang.

"Those warm and genial days of Spring lead up to the heat of Summer, and the anger one might feel in Fall makes way to forgiveness and mercy which one feels in Winter. This change of the four seasons influences the upper and lower pulses.

"To regulate the interior is in accordance with Spring; to have within the right pattern of conduct is in accordance with Summer; to submit to authority is in accordance with Fall; and in accordance with Winter is to weigh inherent rights.

"Winter lasts for forty-five days, and during that time the influence of Yang, the element of light and life, is weak in the upper pulse and the influence of Yin is weak in the lower pulse.

"Summer lasts for forty-five days, and during that time the influence of Yin is weak in the upper pulse and the influence of Yang is weak in the lower pulse.

"Yin and Yang have their respective periods during which they influence the pulse. From the assistance they give each other during this period one can know the functions of the pulse. These functions fall into certain periods, and thus one is able to know the date of death.

"If it were not for excellent technique and the subtlety of the pulse one would not be able to examine it. But the examination must be done according to a plan, and the system of Yin and Yang [the two principles of nature] serves as basis for examination. When this basis is established one can investigate the twelve main vessels and the five elements that generate life. Life itself follows a pattern that was set by the four seasons.

"In order to effect a cure and relief one must not err towards the laws of Heaven nor towards those of the Earth, for they form a unit. When this feeling for Heaven and Earth as one unit has been attained, then one is able to know death as well as life.

"One must understand that music consists of five notes, that physical appearance is made of the five elements, and that the pulse consists of Yin and Yang. Thus one can know that when Yin is flourishing then there occur dreams, as if one had to wade through great waters, which cause bad fears; when Yang is flourishing there occur dreams of great fires which burn and cauterize. When Yin and Yang both are flourishing there occur dreams in which both forces destroy and kill each other or wound each other. When the upper pulse flourishes then there are dreams as though one were flying; and when the lower pulse is flourishing there are dreams as though one were falling down. When one is replete with food then one dreams that one gave up one's inner surplus; when one is hungry or starved then one dreams that one obtained (enough to satisfy one's interior).[4]

"Fullness of the lungs produces dreams of sorrow and weeping. When there is a multitude of small insects then the dreams picture that one has collected all of them. When there is a multitude of large insects then the dreams picture them as clashing together so that they will be injured and destroyed.

"The feeling of the pulse should be done according to method: for when it is slow and quiet it acts as protector and guardian. In days of Spring the pulse is superficial, like wood floating on water (浮) or like a fish that glides through the waves. In Summer days the pulse within the skin is drifting and light (泛 泛), and everywhere there is an excess of creation. In Fall days the torpid insects underneath the skin are about to come out. In Winter the torpid insects are all around the bone, quiet and delicate like the nobleman (君 子) residing in his mansion.

"Hence it is said: Those who wish to know the inner body feel the pulse and have thus the fundamentals for diagnosis.[5] Those who wish to know the exterior of the body observe death and birth.[6] Of these six (the pulse and the five colors) the feeling of the pulse is the most important medium of diagnosis.[7]

4. The part in brackets was added by Wang Ping.
5. Wang Ping explains: To know the interior means to know the pulse and respiration, thus the feeling of the pulse provides the principle of diagnosis.
6. Wang Ping explains: To know the exterior of the body means to know complexion and appearance, therefore they use the five colors for the diagnosis of death and they do the same for the diagnosis of birth.
7. After having looked at these six, one knows the shifting and changing connected with the pulse.

"When the heart pulse beats vigorously (堅) and the strokes are markedly prolonged[8], the corresponding illness makes the tongue curl up and makes the patient unable to speak. When the pulse beats are soft (耎) and scattered like willow blossoms scattering with the wind, it is fitting that one diffuse the encirclement of the corresponding illness.

"When the pulse of the lungs beats vigorously and long, the corresponding illness produces blood in the sputum;[9] when the pulse beats are soft and scattered, the corresponding illness produces torrents of sweat which up till the present time cannot be absorbed and be issued again.

"When the pulse of the liver beats vigorously and long and the complexion is not grayish green, the corresponding illness produces a sinking sensation as though one were fatally stricken, and the blood within the ribs and flanks descends presently, leaving people panting and exhausted. When the pulse beats are soft and scattered and the complexion shining and glossy, the corresponding illness requires abundant drinking, thirst is violent and requires more drinking, and changes befall the flesh and the skin and are transmitted to the outside through the stomach and the bowels.

"When the pulse of the stomach beats vigorously and long, the complexion turns red and the corresponding illness causes bent or broken thighs. When the pulse beats are soft and scattered, the resulting illness causes great pains while eating food.[10]

"When the pulse of the spleen beats vigorously and long and the complexion turns yellow, the corresponding illness produces a shortness of breath and reduced force of life. When the pulse beats are soft and scattered and the complexion is not glossy and shining, the corresponding illness produces swelling of the coccyx and of the feet, which assume the appearance as though they contained water.

"When the pulse of the kidneys beats vigorously and long and the complexion is yellow and red, the corresponding illness produces a bowed posture (折 腰). When the pulse beats are soft and scattered, the resulting illness causes a reduction of blood which is then unable to move."

8. Wang Ping explains: "at the pulse of the hand."
9. Wang Ping explains: When the lungs are completely exhausted, the *lo* (絡) vessels rebel and emit blood, which is secreted with the sputum.
10. Wang Ping explains that 痹 "numbness" should read 痛 "painful."

The Emperor said: "When one examines the pulse of the heart and finds it hasty, what sickness is then indicated? And what form does this illness take?"

Ch'i Po answered: "The name of the disease is 'rupture of the heart' (心疝)[11], and it is in the small intestines[12] where the disease becomes visible."

The Emperor asked: "How can you describe the disease?"

Ch'i Po answered: "The heart acts as bolt of the door to the store-house; the small intestines act as messengers; therefore one says that the small intestines are the place where the disease becomes manifest."

The Emperor inquired: "When, upon examination, one finds that the pulse of the stomach indicates disease, what does then happen?"

Ch'i Po answered: "When the pulse of the stomach is full and slightly tense (實) it indicates dropsical swellings; when it is empty slow and compressible (虛) it indicates a leakage."

The Emperor asked: "How can one describe the process of falling ill and the changes it brings about?"

Ch'i Po responded: "It is the winds and the weather (the eight winds) that cause chills and the fevers. Diseases arising from over-work (癉) cause exhaustion of the diaphragm.[13] Oppressive airs[14] cause madness; constant winds cause inability to retain food;[15] and when abundant winds cause diseases within the pulse they bring about sores and ulcers. The transformations and changes wrought by illness cannot be overcome or even enumerated."

The Emperor inquired: "All sorts of ulcers and swellings, of contracted muscles and aching bones, can they be soothed and can life yet be preserved?"

Ch'i Po replied: "The swellings caused by frost belong to the changes brought about by the eight winds."

The Emperor asked: "How can they be cured?"

Ch'i Po answered: "They belong to the diseases caused by the four seasons; they can be overcome and treated and improvement can be achieved."

11. This term has now come to mean angina pectoris.
12. Wang Ping equals 少腹 to 小腸, the small intestines.
13. Wang Ping explains: "Although the people eat well they remain very thin."
14. Wang Ping explains 厥 to mean 氣逆, oppressive airs or contrary weather.
15. Wang Ping explains: "Food remains undigested and thus leaks out."

The Emperor asked: "What is the cause of these diseases? Is it that the five viscera issue these diseases which injure the pulse and the color (色 complexion)? And should one not know the length, the gravity and the possible result of each disease?"

Ch'i Po answered: "Yes, one must understand all this. This is an excellent question! When there is proof that the pulse is reduced and that the complexion is not violated, then the disease is a recent one. But when there is proof that the pulse is not discordant yet the complexion is affected, then the disease is chronic. When there is proof that the pulse and the five colors (of the complexion) are all equally disturbed, then again the disease is chronic. When upon investigation it is found that the pulse and the five colors are equally undisturbed, then the disease is of recent date.

"When the pulses of the liver and the kidneys coincide and the related colors are azure and red, the corresponding disease has a destructive and injurious power. The blood that was invisible comes to an end and the blood that was visible is so liquefied that it gives the impression as if it were flowing through water.

"The inner pulses in the arms[16] both denote the state of adjacent regions; they denote the state of the short ribs (季 脅). The outer pulses of the arms denote the state of the kidneys. When the pulses of the arms are examined for the interior, they indicate that which goes on within the stomach. Furthermore, the left outer pulse of the arm denotes the state of the liver, while the left inner pulse indicates the state of the diaphragm.[17] The right outer pulse denotes the condition of the stomach and the right inner pulse indicates the state of the spleen. Moreover, the upper right pulse of the outside denotes what goes on within the thorax, whereas the upper left pulse of the outside denotes the condition of the heart and the upper left pulse of the inside indicates what goes on within the middle of the thorax.

"The front is examined for information about the condition of the front. The back is examined in order to obtain information about the condition of the back. Before the examination is completed[18], the state of the thorax and the interior of the throat are examined,

16. Wang Ping equals 尺 丙 to 尺 澤 之 丙.
17. 鬲 translated as 膈.
18. Wang Ping writes 上 竟 上 者 as 上 音 上 至 and 下 音 下, which might be translated as "Rising and falling tones."

and to finish up the examination one probes into the condition of the small intestines, the waist and the loins, the thighs, the knees, and the shinbones.

"When the pulse is dense and coarse and large its content of Yin elements is insufficient, and there is a surplus of Yang elements which causes fevers within the body.

"When an illness has arrived and departs very slowly and the upper pulse is full and large and the lower pulse is empty and slow, these symptoms indicate madness. When the disease which has arrived slowly departs and when the upper pulse is slow and empty, and the lower pulse is full and large, it indicates evil influences. Thus it is found that Yang suffers evil influences within the body.

"When the pulse beats are heavy the examiner should make a careful count, for the (the region of the) lesser Yin is rebellious. When the pulse beats are heavy and upon careful examination are found to be scattered and irregular, they indicate chills and fevers. When the pulse beats are light and floating and also scattered and irregular, they indicate dizziness and blurred vision and people are apt to fall down prostrate.

"When the pulse beats are all light and floating and not hasty, then they all stem from the (region of) Yang and thus they indicate fever.

"When the pulse beats are small and heavy then they all stem from (the region of) Yin and thus they indicate aching bones. When the pulse is calm and quiet the disease is indicated by the pulse of the foot.

"When for a stretch of time the disease is indicated by the pulse of Yang, urine and stool which are secreted contain pus and blood.

"All those who excel in the art of feeling the pulse find that when it is fine, slow, and short, there is an excess of Yang and when the pulse is slippery, like pebbles rolling in a basin, there is an excess of Yin.

"When there is an excess of Yang the body is hot and feverish and there is no perspiration. When there is an excess of Yin there is too much perspiration and colds and chills.

"When one feels at the inside the pulse which indicates the outside, and when this inside pulse does not indicate the outside, there is a (harmful) accumulation within the heart and the stomach.

"When one feels at the outside the pulse which indicates the inside, and when it does not indicate the inside, the body is hot and feverish.

"When one feels the pulse at the highest point and it does not descend, it means that the loins and the feet are emaciated (in a poor condition). When one feels the pulse at the lowest point and it does not ascend, it means that there is an ache within the head and the neck.

"When at the end of the examination of the pulse the strength of the pulse of the bones is small, it is indicated that the loins and the spine ache and that the body suffers from numbness."

18. *Treatise on the Manifestations of Health in Man*

The Yellow Emperor asked: "What constitutes a healthy person?"

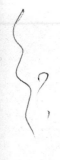

Ch'i Po answered: "Man has one exhalation to one pulse beat which is then repeated, and he has one inhalation to one pulse beat which is also repeated. Exhalation and inhalation determine the beat of the pulse. When there are five respiratory movements to one pulse beat, it means that there is one extra movement inserted, bringing about a deep breath (太息) of what is called a healthy and well-balanced person. A healthy and well-balanced person is not affected by disease.

"Those who are habitually without disease help to train and to adjust those who are sick, for those who treat should be free from illness. Therefore they train the patient to adjust his breathing, and in order to train the patient, they act as example.

"When a person has one exhalation to three movements of the pulse and one inhalation to three movements of the pulse, and when the 'cubit' (尺) indicates fever, one speaks of it as the 'warm sickness.' When the 'cubit' is not hot and the pulse is slippery one speaks of a sickness caused by the winds (the eight motivating powers). When the pulse beats are small, fine and slow, one speaks of numbness.

"When a person has one exhalation to four movements of the pulse above, it means that death will follow. When the pulse breaks off and does not extend it also means death. When the pulse gets abruptly disconnected, or accelerates suddenly, it means death. Uninterrupted and regular breathing is to a healthy person what a granary is to the stomach, [i.e.] it is the stomach which causes a healthy person's regular breathing and steady constitution. If a person has no breath in his stomach he is described as being in disorder, and those who are in disorder must die.

"In Spring (the pulse) of the stomach should be fine and delicate like the strings of a musical instrument. If the strings are touched too frequently, the stomach functions intermittently and the resulting illness affects the liver. If the strings give only one tone the stomach ceases to function and death results. When the stomach has a defect an illness will make its appearance in harvest time. When the defect or idiosyncracy is great the illness will strike at once.

"The viscera thoroughly expel into the liver. Thus the liver harbors the force of life of the muscles and the thin membranes.

"In Summer the pulse of the stomach should be like the beats of a fine hammer; then it is healthy and well-balanced. When the hammer beats are too heavy the stomach works insufficiently and an illness of the heart results. When there is only one single hammer beat the stomach has ceased to function and death ensues. When the stomach contains stones a disease will make its appearance in Winter. When the stones are large the disease will break out presently. The viscera are in thorough communication and bound by circulation with the heart, and the blood that is stored by the heart, and thus the blood fills the pulse with the force of life (breath).

"During the long Summer (長夏) the pulse of the stomach should be soft and feeble; then it is healthy and well-balanced. But when it is too feeble, the stomach functions insufficiently and an illness of the spleen results. When the pulse is soft and feeble and there are also stones (in the stomach), a disease will make its appearance in Winter. When the pulse is of great weakness the disease breaks out presently.

"The viscera fill the spleen with moisture. Thus the spleen harbors the force of life of the flesh.

"In Autumn the pulse of the stomach should be small and rough; then it is healthy and well-balanced. But when it is too rough the stomach functions insufficiently and a disease of the lungs results. When it is merely rough death results. When it is rough but also taut like the strings of a lute, a disease will make its appearance in Spring. When the pulse beats resemble too closely the tautness of musical strings a disease breaks out presently. The lungs are the highest of the five viscera, and make the blood and the vital essences circulate freely, guarding and protecting Yin and Yang [the principles of life and death].

"In Winter the pulse of the stomach should be small and like stone; then it is healthy and well-balanced. When it is too much like a stone the stomach functions insufficiently and a disease of the kidneys results. When it sounds like a single stone the stomach ceases to function and death ensues. When it is stone-like but also like the beating of a hammer, a disease will make its appearance in Summer. When the sound that is comparable to the beating of a hammer is too strong, the disease will develop at once.

"The lowest of the viscera are the kidneys, thus the kidneys harbor the force of life of the bones and the marrow.

"The great arteries (*lo vessels*) of the stomach are described as 'hollow lanes' creating a connection with the vessels of the lungs, which descend along the left breast. The motion of these vessels corresponds[1] to that of the pulse in the support of the force of life. When there is much coughing and troubled breathing the breath is frequently interrupted, and then an illness within the stomach will develop, causing coagulation and irritation through an accumulation (of food); this will never be able to pass through, and death will result. The motion of the vessels underneath the breast serve to support the force of life and to keep it from leaking out.

"And now one should turn to the discussion of the effect which is caused by an excess of the 'inch' pulse (寸 口) and of the effect when it is inadequate. When the 'inch' pulse within the hand is short and without volume (短), a headache results. When the 'inch' pulse within the hand is too much prolonged extreme pains on feet and shinbones result.[2] When the 'inch' pulse within the hand routs and strikes upward, the result is a shoulder and back ache. When the 'inch' pulse at the wrist is deep, like a stone thrown into water (沈) and also vigorous, an illness within the body results. When the 'inch' pulse is superficial like a piece of wood floating upon water (浮) and abundant, then an illness of the external body results.

"When the 'inch' pulse is deep and yet feeble, there will be chills and fevers and even rupture of the bowels (疝 瘕) and pains of the

---

1. 衣 is here translated as 依.
2. Wang Ping explains: The shortness of the pulse indicates that Yang cannot penetrate and this causes a headache; a prolonged pulse indicates that there is an excess of Yin causing sore feet.

small intestines. When the 'inch' pulse is deep and yet violent, it means that there is a congestion under the ribs and that within the stomach there is an evil accumulation located crosswise, which causes pains. When the 'inch' pulse is deep and there is shortness of breath, it indicates chills and fevers. When the pulse is abundant and slippery (滑) and also vigorous, it is said that the disease affects the external body; when the pulse is small, long and slightly tense (實) and also vigorous, the disease affects the internal body. When the pulse is small, weak and therefore very fine, slow and short (濇), it indicates a chronic disease. When the pulse is slippery and superficial and also hasty, it indicates a new disease.

"When the pulse is irritated (急) it means that there exists a difficulty in breathing and pains in the small intestines. When the pulse is slippery it means that the eight winds are at work, and when the pulse is small and fine it means that there is numbness. When the pulse is tardy like willow branches swaying to a light breeze, and slippery, like pebbles rolling in a basin, it means that there are fevers raging within the body. When the pulse is abundant but tense and hard and full like a cord (緊), there are dropsical swellings.

"When the pulse beats in accord with Yin and Yang, the disease changes for the better and comes to an end; but when the pulse beats are in opposition to Yin and Yang the disease becomes worse. When the pulse obediently follows the four seasons there will be no disease; but when the pulse does not beat in consonance with the four seasons it will not extend to the regions between the five viscera and the resulting disease will be difficult to cure. When the arms are prone to be of a greenish-gray color it is said that the pulse is drained of blood.

"When the 'cubit' pulse is slow and tardy and small, it is said to be loosening and dissolving and improving (体). When a person lies down very quietly while the pulse is abundant, it indicates that the body is drained of blood. When the 'cubit' pulse is small and the pulse in general is slippery, the indication is that there is an excess of blood. When the 'cubit' pulse is cold and the pulse in general is slender, the indication is given that there is a leakage in the patient's posterior. When the pulse [in general] and the 'cubit' pulse [in particular] are coarse and rough and there is constant heat, the indication is given that there are fevers within the body.

"When in relation to the liver the celestial stems *kêng hsin* 庚 辛

become visible it means death.³   When in relation to the heart the celestial stems *jên kuei* 壬 癸 appear it means death.⁴   When in relation to the spleen the celestial stems *chia i* 甲 乙 become visible it means death.⁵   When in relation to the lungs the celestial stems *ping ting* 丙 丁 become visible it means death.⁶   When in relation to the kidneys the celestial stems *wu chi* 戊 己 become visible it means death.⁷   All this means that the viscera can all cause death.

"When the motion of the pulse of the neck (is abundant⁸) coughing and troubled breathing occur, and this is said to have been caused through water.⁹   When within the eye there is a minute swelling, as though a dormant silkworm were beginning to take shape, it is said to have been caused through water.¹⁰   When the urine is reddish yellow, although the patient rests quietly, it indicates jaundice and ulcers (黃 疸).¹¹   When a person has just finished eating and yet feels hungry stomach ulcers are indicated.   When the face swells it is caused by winds;¹² when feet and knees swell it is caused by water. When the eye turns yellow it is called jaundice.

"The hand of woman belongs to the region of lesser Yin.   When the motion of her pulse is great she is with child.   The pulse has ways of indicating whether the patient follows or disobeys the laws of the four seasons and whether there are or are not hidden symptoms; for instance, when in Spring and Summer the pulse is thin (瘦) and when in Fall and Winter the pulse is superficial (浮) and large, it is clearly indicated that the patient is in discord with the four seasons.

"Even when there is a disease and fever, the pulse can nevertheless be quiet and still; and even when there is a leakage and much blood is lost the pulse can nevertheless be full and large.   The disease

---

3. Wang Ping explains: the celestial stems 庚 辛 stand for the element of metal, but the liver is connected with the element of wood.

4. Wang Ping explains: the celestial stems 壬 癸 stand for the element of water, but the heart is connected with the element of fire.

5. Wang Ping explains: the celestial stems 甲 乙 stand for the element of wood, while the spleen is connected with the element of the earth.

6. Wang Ping explains: the celestial stems 丙 丁 stand for the element of fire, while the lungs are connected with the element of metal.

7. Wang Ping explains: 戊 己 stands for the element of earth, while the kidneys are connected with the element of water.

8. The words in parentheses were added in the commentary by Wang Ping.

9. Wang Ping explains: "Through the rising vapors of the water."

10. Wang Ping explains: "Through water within the stomach."

11. Wang Ping explains: "This trouble is caused through illness of the kidneys and fever within the bladder."

12. Wang Ping adds: "Winds within the stomach."

is within when the pulse is empty and slow, and the disease is at the outside when the pulse is small and fine and yet vigorous. All these diseases are difficult to treat and to cure, for they are known to be caused by opposition to the laws of the four seasons. Man uses water and grain as his basis of existence, hence when he is without water and grain he must die. When the pulse is not reinforced by the stomach man must also die. Those pulses which are not reinforced by the stomach merely obtain the support of the viscera, but not the vital force of the stomach. Those people who are deprived of the vital force of the stomach have a pulse of the liver that is not taut like a musical string (弦), and a pulse of the kidneys that is not coarse and rough like a stone (石).

"The pulses of the regions of the lesser Yin sound near at first, but then they change abruptly to more distant sounds; they are short at first and then they change suddenly to longer sounds.

"The pulses of the regions of the 'sunlight' are superficial and large and also short and without volume; they strike the finger sharply and leave it quickly.

"When man is serene and healthy the pulse of the heart flows and connects, just as pearls are joined together or like a string of red jade—then one can speak of a healthy heart.

"In summer the life-giving force of the stomach is regarded as the origin of life.

"When man is sick the pulse of his heart rushes and pants. When this panting is continuous and springs from within and the pulse beats are wrong and small—then one can speak of a sick heart.

"At the point of death the pulse of the heart flows in front but is faulty and feeble in back, and then it stands still as if restrained by a belt or a hook—and then one can speak of the death of the heart.

"When man is tranquil and healthy his pulse of the lungs comes calm and peaceful. And when it is peaceful like a village, or the seeds of an elm tree—then one can speak of healthy lungs.

"In Fall the life-giving force of the stomach is considered the source of life.

"When man is sick the pulse of his lungs moves, but it neither rises nor falls like the wings of a chicken—and then one can speak of sick lungs.

"At the point of death the pulse of the lungs moves like an object that is floating and insubstantial, or like a hair blown by the wind— and then one can speak of the death of the lungs.

"When man is tranquil and healthy the pulse of his liver beats softly and weakly, as if one sounded a long thin bamboo rod without a tip—and then one can speak of a healthy liver.

"In Spring the life-giving force of the stomach is considered the foundation of life.

"When man is sick the pulse of the liver moves fully, and it is large and long and slightly tense, felt on both light and heavy pressure; but it is also slippery like the sound of many long bamboo rods strung together, and then one can speak of a sick liver.

"At the point of death the pulse of the liver moves with increased speed and strength, like a new long bow of a musical instrument—and then one can speak of the death of the liver.

"When man is tranquil and healthy the pulse of the spleen flows softly, coming together and falling apart like a chicken treading the earth—and then one can speak of a healthy spleen.

"In Summer the life-giving force of the stomach is considered the basis of life.

"When man is sick the pulse of the spleen moves fully and is large and long and slightly tense, and there is a surplus of the number of pulse beats like a chicken raising its feet—and then one can speak of a sick spleen.

"At the point of death the pulse of the spleen moves sharply and strongly like the beak of a bird, or like the spurs of a cock, or like the leakage of a house, or even like torrents of water—and then one can speak of the death of the spleen.

"When man is tranquil and healthy the pulse of the kidneys flows as though it were panting and weary, as though it were alternately repressed and connected and very firm—and then one can speak of healthy kidneys.

"In Winter the life-giving force of the stomach is considered the origin of life.

"When man is ill the pulse of the kidneys flows like the sound that is made by touching the stretched fibres of beans[13] and its strength is increased;—and then one can speak of sick kidneys.

"At the point of death the pulse of the kidneys flows and makes itself manifest like the tearing of twisted cord or like the snapping of fingers upon stone—and then one can speak of the death of the kidneys."

13. Wang Ping says: "The shape of the kidneys is then like the stretched fibres of a bean."

Book 6

19. Treatise on the Precious Mechanism of the Viscera

THE Yellow Emperor asked: "In Spring the pulse is like the strings of a lute; why is this the case?"

Ch'i Po answered: "In Spring the pulse is that of the liver; and wood is the element of the East. Spring is the time of the beginning of the creation of all living beings; therefore their breath is still flowing softly and weakly, their pulse is slow and slippery, but they keep themselves upright and straight and are in the process of growing, and therefore one compares them to the strings of a lute. When the condition is the opposite then they are sick."

The Emperor asked: "How could the opposite of these conditions come about?"

Ch'i Po answered: "If their breath moves deeply and strongly, one would call this excess and beyond proper limits, and disease is bound to arise upon their exterior. But if their breath does not come deeply but delicately, one can say that it is inadequate and that the disease has reached the interior of the body."

The Emperor inquired: "What does happen when there is an excess of pulse action in Spring? Will disease then attack the entire system?"

Ch'i Po answered: "Excess causes man to forget what is proper and good and he becomes careless. Carelessness dazes him so that he walks as though his eyes were covered and he falls prey to madness. And even if this does not happen, he will get pains in his thorax which bend his back downwards, affecting both his flanks and his armpits."

The Emperor asked: "Should not the pulse in Summer be like a hammer or can it sound different from a hammer?"

Ch'i Po answered: "In Summer the pulse is that of the heart; and fire is the element of the South. All things in creation flourish and grow, therefore the breath of all living creatures is plentiful in coming, and decreases in leaving, and thus it is said to be like a hammer. When the condition is the opposite then they are sick."

The Emperor said: "How could the opposite of these conditions come about?"

Ch'i Po answered: "If their breath comes in plentifully and leaves just as plentifully, then one would call this excess and beyond proper limits, and disease would arise upon their exterior. But if their breath does not come plentifully and leaves in the opposite condition, then one can say that it is insufficient and that the disease has reached the interior of the body."

The Emperor asked: "What will happen when there is an excess of pulse action in Summer? Will the disease then affect the entire system?"

Ch'i Po answered: "Excess causes man's body to be hot and his skin and flesh to ache; his body will gradually be flooded and unable to live, he will have heart trouble; coughing and spitting will make their appearance above, while below the breath of life is caused to leak out."

The Emperor asked: "Is it not regular that i.. Fall the pulse should be superficial and flowing, light like a piece of wood floating on water—or can it be other than superficial?"

Ch'i Po answered: "In Fall the pulse is that of the lungs; and metal is the element of the West. All things in creation approach their harvest, perfection and completion. Therefore the breath flows lightly and the pulse is slow and superficial. Since the breath comes quickly and scatters when leaving, one can say that it is superficial. If the condition is the opposite then one can say that there is sickness."

The Emperor said: "How could the opposite of these conditions come about?"

Ch'i Po replied: "If the breath comes roughly and the heart beats vigorously while they are both depending upon a slow pulse, then one would call this excess and disease would arise upon the exterior. But if the breath comes roughly and is nevertheless feeble, it means that it is inadequate and that the disease has reached the interior of the body."

The Emperor asked: "What will happen when there is an excess of pulse action in Fall? Will then disease affect the entire system?"

Ch'i Po answered: "Excess causes man to have trouble while breathing, and consequently his back will hurt badly, he will be in pain and have fevers which make him unfit for life. He will be obliged to pant while inhaling and exhaling, and because the force of his breath is reduced he will cough. One can find that above blood is secreted with his breath, and below one can perceive the typical sounds of illness."

The Emperor asked: "Should not in Winter the pulse be well regulated or could it be other than well regulated?"

Ch'i Po answered: "In Winter the pulse is that of the kidneys; and water is the element of the North. All things in creation live shut in and (the crop) is stored away. Therefore the breath comes from deep within and strikes out strongly, and thus it is said to be well regulated. When the condition is the opposite man is sick."

The Emperor asked: "How could the opposite of these conditions come about?"

Ch'i Po answered: "If the breath comes like the snapping of fingers upon stone one would call this excess, and disease would arise upon their exterior. But if the breath comes too frequently, then it is inadequate; it means that the disease has reached the interior of the body."

The Emperor inquired: "What will happen when there is an excess of pulse action in Winter? Will the disease affect the entire system?"

Ch'i Po replied: "Excess causes man to relax his spine and his pulse action, and he will be in pain. And since his breathing capacity is reduced he does not have a desire to speak, and this makes him unfit (for living), causing him to be in anxious suspense, which is similar to a disease. Dearth and hunger rage within his ribs, there is fasting within his spine and pains within his small intestines, and although man is full there is little transformation into urine."

The Emperor said: "These are suitable (explanations)" and then he went on to say, "Obedience or disobedience to the order of the four seasons brings about either change or calamity. Yet how can you control the pulse of the spleen when it acts independently from the others?"

Ch'i Po answered: "The pulse of the spleen is connected with the element of the earth. The spleen is a solitary organ, but it can irrigate the four others[1] that are nearby."

The Emperor asked: "But how can one perceive whether the spleen is in an excellent or in an evil condition?"

1. Wang Ping explains the four others to be liver, heart, lungs, and kidneys.

Ch'i Po answered: "When the spleen is in an excellent condition there is nothing that can be perceived, but when it is in an evil condition it can be easily seen."

The Emperor asked: "But how can it be seen that it is in an evil condition?"

Ch'i Po answered: "Then the pulse of the spleen beats like the unstable drifting of water, and it can be described as excessive; and disease has befallen the exterior of the body. But when it sounds like the pecking of the beak of a bird, then it is insufficient and the disease has penetrated into the interior of the body."

The Emperor said: "The master (夫 子) has described the spleen as acting as a solitary organ, located in the center like the earth, and irrigating the four organs that are located nearby. When the spleen works excessively, it is inadequate; will then all the organs be affected by disease?"

Ch'i Po replied: "Excess causes man to be unable to lift his four limbs, and this inadequacy brings about that the nine orifices of his body no longer communicate with each other; and then one says that the impulse of the viscera has become either heavy or violent."

The Emperor was startled and then he rose, paid homage repeatedly, and bowed to the ground; then he said: "How excellent that I now know the essentials of the pulse, the final destiny of everything below Heaven, the five colors, and that the changes which the pulse might undergo can be calculated and prefigured. And it is strange and wonderful that Tao, the right way, is in each of them and combines them into one entity.

"When the spiritual powers are passed on and transmitted they can no longer turn back; and when they turn back they cannot be transmitted, and then their moving powers are lost to the universe. In order to fulfil destiny man should go beyond that which is near at hand and consider it as trifling. One should make public upon tablets of jade that which was hidden and concealed in treasuries and storehouses, to study it from early dawn until night, and thus make known the precious mechanism of the universe.[2]

"The five viscera receive the impact of the life-giving force from those who generate them, and they pass it on to those whom they subjugate. Their force of life is bestowed upon those whom they

2. 著 之 玉 版 藏 之 藏 府 每 旦 讀 之 名 曰 玉 機.

beget, but they bring death upon those who cannot overcome their diseases. Moreover, death naturally takes preference in summoning those who have reached the state where they cannot overcome their diseases and must thus die. This means that living in opposition to the breath of life brings about death.

"When the liver receives the life-giving force (氣) from the heart, it is from there transmitted to the spleen, whence it is passed on to the kidneys; here it reaches its utmost, so that it meets death when it arrives at the lungs.

"When the heart receives the life-giving force from the spleen, it is from there transmitted to the lungs, then it is passed on to the liver; here it reaches its utmost, so that it meets death when it arrives at the kidneys.

"When the spleen receives the life-giving force from the lungs, it is from there transmitted to the kidneys, thence it is passed on to the heart; here it reaches its utmost, so that it meets death when it arrives at the liver.

"When the lungs receive the life-giving force from the kidneys, it is from there transmitted to the liver, thence it is passed on to the spleen; here it reaches its utmost, so that it meets death when it arrives at the heart.

"When the kidneys receive the life-giving force from the liver, it is from there transmitted to the heart, and thence passed on to the lungs; here it reaches its utmost, so that it meets death when it arrives at the spleen.

"All this is death brought about by unnatural procedure.[3] After the observation of one day and one night and their five divisions (五 分),[4] one can foretell death and life and whether death will strike early or whether life will last long."

The Emperor said: "The five viscera are in communication with one another and influence one another, and each of the five viscera has one that is secondary to it. When the five viscera are sick then each passes it on to that which is inferior. When one does not know the method for treatment and cure, then three months are like six months and they are like three days or six days, it will spread over the five viscera and death will follow, for it is in accordance (with nature) that the disease will be transferred to those viscera that are

3. 此 皆 逆 死 也.
4. Wang Ping explains those to be the five combinations of the celestial stems.

inferior and next in order.   Therefore it is said that one must distinguish between [the three regions of Yang] and be aware of their
diseases from the beginning; and one must distinguish between [the
three regions of] Yin in order to know the dates of life and death.
This means to say that one can know the limit of the weariness of
the viscera and their consequent death.[5]

"The (evil) winds contribute to the development of a hundred
diseases.[6]   When the present wind is cold and it strikes man, it will
cause his body hair to stand out straight and it will cause his skin
to be stopped up, and man will become hot and feverish (熱).   At
that time he can perspire and thus send forth (the evil influences
within).[7]   But it is also possible that numbness brings about swellings and pains.   At that time one must apply hot liquids and hot
irons and finally resort to fire, which is used in burning moxa for
cauterization, and thus bring about the disappearance (of the evil
winds).

"If one does not treat this disease it will enter (the body) and
reside at the lungs, and then its name is numbness of the lungs, which
emit a cough of the upper respiratory tract.   If one does not treat
the lungs then the disease will spread forthwith and will affect the
liver,   causing   a   disease   called   numbness   of   the   liver.   This
name also indicates that there are pains within the flanks at the
intake of food.   If at the same time one should find that the ear is
irritated, and if this is not treated, the liver passes the disease on to
the spleen.   The name of the (resulting) disease means that the
(evil) influences (winds 風) of the spleen create a feeling of hunger
even after one has eaten, weariness (癉), and a burning sensation
within the stomach, an irritation of the heart, and the complexion
will turn yellow.[8]

"At that time one can repress the disease, one can administer
drugs and one can apply baths.   But if these treatments do not
bring about a cure the spleen will transmit the disease to the kidneys.
The name of the resulting disease is hernia (rupture) of the bowels
(疝 瘕).   The small intestines are the victims; they are feverish and

5. Wang Ping explains this to mean: "Death for those who can no longer overcome (their
     diseases)."
6. Wang Ping explains: "The evil Winds are the origin of a hundred diseases."
7. The words in brackets were added by Wang Ping.
8. 色 was added by Wang Ping.

afflicted with pains and white secretions[9] make their appearance. The name of this disease also indicates dropsy (swellings).

"Now one can repress the disease and can administer drugs. If a cure is not achieved the kidneys will pass on the disease to the heart. The muscles (sinews, nerves 筋) and the arteries (veins, pulse 脉) will disunite from each other and an acute illness will develop, which is called 'convulsions' (瘛＝瘲?).[10] When at that time neither cauterization by burning moxa nor the application of drugs brings about a cure, then even after suitable treatment of fully ten days death will occur.

"For, after the kidneys have infected the heart, the heart forthwith returns the infection and passes it on to the lungs, where it becomes manifest by chills and fevers; and death follows after three years. This is how the diseases strike the organs which are next in order. But those diseases which end suddenly after having spread must not necessarily have been treated. Or, perhaps, when they were spread and underwent changes, there were no more secondary (organs). And when there are no more secondary organs in which to enter, then (the five emotions): grief (憂), fear (恐), pity (悲), joy (喜), and anger (怒) cannot change into those that are secondary to them and thus cause man to become gravely ill.

"Hence, when joy is felt it creates a large vacuum (大 虛), and thus the force of the kidneys can ascend.[11] The emotion of anger arises from the fullness of the liver. The emotion of sympathy arises from the fullness of the lungs. The emotion of fear releases the impulses of the spleen.[12] The feeling of worry releases the impulses of the heart.[13]

"These are the ways of the emotions, and thus disease has five times five, twenty-five, possible transformations until it can be

9. 液 was added by Wang Ping.
10. Wang Ping explains: "When the kidneys do not work sufficiently, then no water is generated; consequently the muscles become parched, dry, and convulsed and therefore disunite from each other."
11. Wang Ping explains: "Joy is the emotion of the heart which then influences the lungs, leaving the heart unprotected; thus the influences of the kidneys are permitted to come to the fore."
12. Wang Ping explains: "Fear is the emotion of the kidneys, and influences the heart, leaving the kidneys unprotected; thus the influences of the spleen are permitted to come to the fore."
13. Wang Ping explains: "Sadness is the emotion of the liver, and influences the spleen, leaving the liver unprotected; thus the influences of the heart come to the fore."

passed on and changed again.   To spread a disease (傳) means to release it, to multiply it, or to have it come to the fore (乘).

"When man grows old his bones become dry (and brittle like) straw and his flesh sags (陷).   Within his thorax there is much air, resulting in panting and troubled breathing; when he then cannot ease nature and be rid of his vapors and move his bowels, his body will die within a period of six months.   But if this becomes evident by the pulse of the lungs,[14] the period granted is only one day.

"When man grows old his bones become dry and brittle like straw, his flesh sags and there is much gas within his thorax, resulting in panting and troubled breathing.   When he then cannot ease nature he gets pains within his body.   Then the top of his shoulders and the nape of his neck contract, and death occurs within a period of one month.   But when this becomes noticeable by (the pulse of) the heart,[15] the period granted is only one day.

"When man grows old his bones become dry and brittle like straw and his flesh sags and there is much gas within his thorax, resulting in panting and troubled breathing.   When he then cannot ease nature, and has pains within, and when the top of his shoulders and the nape of his neck are contracted, when his body burns with fever and his bones are stripped (of the flesh) and laid bare, his condition will become visible (by the pulse of) the spleen,[15] and death will strike at the interior of the body within a period of ten months.

"When man grows old his bones become dry and brittle like straw, his flesh sags, the marrow within his bones disintegrates, and his movements deteriorate increasingly; when then the (pulse of the) kidneys[16] is about to become noticeable, death will strike within one year; but if (the pulse of the kidneys) has become noticeable the allotted span is but one day.

"When man grows old his bones become dry and brittle like straw, his flesh sags and there is much air within his thorax, and pains within his stomach; there is an uncomfortable feeling within his heart, the nape of his neck and the top of his shoulders (are contracted), his body burns with fever, his bones are stripped and laid bare of flesh, and his eyes bulge and sag.   When then the (pulse of the) liver[16] can be seen but the eye can no longer recognize a raphe, death will strike.

14. Wang Ping explains 眞 藏 to mean: lungs, heart, spleen.
15. Wang Ping explains 眞 藏 to mean: lungs, heart, spleen.
16. Wang Ping explains 眞 藏 to mean: kidneys and liver.

The limit of man's life can be perceived when man can no longer overcome (his diseases); then his time of death has arrived.

"Haste and emptiness within the body arrive suddenly. The five viscera are interrupted in their work and become stopped up; the ways of the pulse no longer function and circulate. Breath does not go in and come out, it is—to use a simile—like falling and being given over to sinking, and there is no time left at all.[17] The pulses are interrupted and do not flow, as though man were one with death. The breath[18] comes five or six times and then man's physical shape has ceased to exist; the flesh has ceased to sag, but although the pulses of the viscera cannot be perceived it is doubtful whether he is dead.

"When the pulse of the liver stops there is anxiety within and at the outside of the body, as though man were followed by the punishing edge of a sword that were charging blazingly, or as though guitars and lutes were pressed down. The complexion turns green and white and loses its glossy appearance, the body hair breaks off and death strikes.

"When the pulse of the heart ceases to beat firmly and becomes weary like the seeds of 'Job's tears' (coix lachryma), the complexion turns red and black and loses its glossy appearance, the body hair breaks off and death strikes.

"When the pulse of the lungs stops its large and slow beats and (sounds) as though there were hair and feathers, the complexion of the human skin turns white and red and loses its glossy appearance, the body hair breaks off and death strikes.

"When the pulse of the kidneys stops beating and becomes interrupted as though fingers were snapped upon stone and swerved, the complexion turns black and yellow and loses its glossy appearance, the body hair breaks off and death strikes.

"When the pulse of the spleen stops beating softly and deeply and increases suddenly and then abruptly decreases, the complexion turns yellow and green and loses its glossy appearance and death strikes.

"All these are the visible symptoms of the viscera, they are all followed by death and cannot be cured."

17. Wang Ping explains 死 日 之 期 to mean: death will strike within the day.
18. Wang Ping says: 息 字 誤 息 當 作 呼 乃 是

The Yellow Emperor asked: "Does it mean death if one perceives the (symptoms) of the viscera?"

Ch'i Po answered: "The five viscera all desire their breath of life from the spleen; it is the spleen that is the foundation of existence of the five viscera.

"The viscera cannot by themselves influence (the pulse of) the hand and (the region of) the great Yin. They must influence the spleen whose vital force then reaches the hand and the region of the great Yin. But each of the five viscera has its special period when it can act by itself and influence the hand and the region of the great Yin.

"When evil influences are victorious, the secretions deteriorate; thus when the disease is grave the vital force of the stomach cannot be entirely given over to (the pulse of) the hand in the region of the great Yin. Under such circumstances the vital force of the viscera only can be perceived, the disease has overpowered the viscera and therefore one speaks of death."

The Emperor exclaimed: "Very well!" and then he said: "To treat and to cure disease means to examine the body, the breath, the complexion, its glossiness or degree of moisture and the pulse, as to whether it is flourishing or deteriorating, and whether the disease is a recent one. But then the actual treatment must follow, for later on there is no time.

"When the vital forces of the body are in mutual agreement it means that cure can be effected. When the complexion and the moisture are excessive the disease can easily be brought to an end. When the pulse is in accord with the four seasons it means that the disease can be cured. When the pulse is feeble and slippery (it is influenced) by the vital forces of the stomach; it means that the disease can be easily cured if one selects the appropriate season.

"When the vital forces of the body are in mutual disagreement one says that the disease is difficult to cure. When the complexion is young but not glossy it means that it is difficult to bring the disease to an end. When the pulse is full and vigorous it means that the disease has become increasingly grave. When the pulse is in discord with the four seasons the disease cannot be cured. With those who are called 'in discord with the four seasons' one can feel their pulse of the lungs in Spring, their pulse of the kidneys in Summer, their pulse of the heart in Fall, and their pulse of the spleen in

Winter,[19] and all these pulses are suspended and interrupted; they are deep, like stones thrown into water, and fine and slow, like scraping bamboo with a knife. And for these reasons they are said to be in discord with the four seasons. There should never be visibility of the viscera. When in Spring and Summer the pulse is deeply impressed and fine and slow, and when in Fall and Winter the pulse is superficial and large, it is said to be in discord with the four seasons, and there will be disease and fever.

"When the pulse is quiet there is a leakage, and when it is large there is a loss of blood; and when the pulse is large and long and slightly tense the disease is within the body. When the pulse is full and large and also vigorous the disease attacks the outside of the body, or the pulse may not be full and vigorous—all these diseases are difficult to cure."

The Yellow Emperor continued: "I understand that the decision of life and death depends upon whether (the pulses) sound hollow or solid. Now I should like to be informed about the circumstances."

Ch'i Po replied: "If the pulses of the five viscera sound (entirely) solid it means death, and if they sound (entirely) hollow it also means death."[20]

The Emperor said: "I should like to be informed about the state of the five viscera when their pulses are either full or hollow."

Ch'i Po answered: "When the pulses are abundant the skin is hot, the stomach is swelled out with dropsy, there is no circulation between front and back, and the center is obscured (閟督＝閟督); then it is said that the five viscera are entirely full of (evil influences).[21]

"When the pulses are slender like a silk thread, the skin is chilled, there is shortness of breath, and what is taken in leaks out in front and in back and food cannot be made to enter. Then it is said that the five viscera are hollow and empty."[22]

19. Instead of the liver in Spring, the heart in Summer, the lungs in Fall, and the kidneys in Winter.
20. Wang Ping explains: 五實五藏之實虛謂五藏虛
21. Wang Ping explains: "實 means 'abundant with evil influences.' The pulse which is abundant with evil influences is that of the heart, the chilled skin belongs to the lungs, an inflated stomach belongs to the spleen, lack of circulation between front and back belongs to the kidneys, and an obscured center belongs to the liver."
22. Wang Ping explains: "虛 means that the vital forces are not sufficient; thus pulses, slender like a silk thread, belong to the heart, the chilled skin belongs to the lungs, the reduced breath belongs to the liver, the kidneys cause all that is gained to leak out, and the spleen prevents both food and drink from being taken in."

The Emperor said: "All those who live have a certain allotted period of life?"

Ch'i Po answered: "When broth and rice gruel enter the stomach and then leak out, one should concentrate upon stopping this condition, for then the viscera become hollow. When the body is active, perspiration can be achieved with advantageous results and then the viscera become full and solid. Thus it is activity that determines the span of life."

20. *Treatise on the Three Regions and the Nine Subdivisions*

The Yellow Emperor said: "In regard to the nine needles (for acupuncture) I understand from the great master that a great many physicians of extensive learning are not able to overcome destiny.[1] I should like to know the requirements of the correct procedure, in order to assemble (this knowledge) so that I can transmit it to my sons and grandsons and make it known to posterity. (I wish to hear about) the bones and the marrow, about the viscera, and about the liver and the lungs.

"I shall smear my mouth with blood and take an oath that I will not venture to receive this information were I to use it recklessly or neglect it.

"I urge you to bring into harmony for me nature, Heaven, and Tao [the right way].[2] There must be an end and a beginning. Heaven must be in accord with the lights of the sky, the celestial bodies, and their course and periods. The earth below must reflect the four seasons, the five elements, that which is precious and that which is lowly and without value—one as well as the other. Is it not that in Winter man responds to Yin [the principle of darkness and cold]? And is it not that in Summer he responds to Yang [the principle of light and warmth]? Let me be informed about their workings."

Ch'i Po replied: "Truly a subtle question! It demands that one decypher Nature (天 地) to the utmost degree."

The Emperor exclaimed: "I should like to be informed about

1. 余 聞 鍼 於 夫 子 衆 多 博 大 不 勝 數.
2. Wang Ping explains that according to 全 元 起 it should read Heaven and Earth (天 地) instead of (天 道) Heaven and Tao.

Nature to the utmost degree and to include (information) about man, his physical form, his blood, his breath of life, his circulation and his dissolution; and I should like to know what causes his death and his life and what we can do about all this."

Ch'i Po answered: "According to the final calculations Nature begins as *one* and ends as *nine*.

"The first is Heaven, the second is Earth, and the third is man. These are the three. Three times three is nine and corresponds to the nine wild regions upon earth.[3]

"Thus man is composed of three parts, and each part has three subdivisions which decide upon life or death. They serve to control the hundred diseases and they serve to blend that which is hollow and solid, that which is abstract and concrete, and thus they fight off noxious influences and diseases."[4]

The Emperor inquired: "How can you explain these three regions?"

Ch'i Po answered: "There is a lower region, there is a middle region, and there is an upper region. Each of these regions has three subdivisions; and within these subdivisions there are contained some elements of Heaven, some elements of Earth, and some elements of Man. One must point this out and teach it in order to achieve the truth.

"The upper regions that contain the elements of Heaven are the arteries (重 脉) upon both sides of the forehead.

"The upper regions that contain the elements of Earth are the arteries within both cheeks (jaws).

"The upper regions that contain the elements of man are the arteries in front of the ears.

"The middle region that contains elements of Heaven is the region of the great Yin, within the hands.[5]

---

3. The *Erh Ya* (爾 雅) says: "Beyond the capital of the district lie the outer suburbs and beyond the suburbs lies the imperial domain. Beyond the imperial domain lie the pastures and beyond the pastures lie the forests and beyond the forests are the border prairies, and beyond the border prairies lie the wild regions (野). This serves to describe their distance."

4. Wang Ping explains: "The so-called three regions are the upper, the middle and the lower part of the body, they do not mean the 'inch' (寸) pulse, the 'bar' (關) pulse, and the 'cubit' (尺) pulse . . . and because of this the help rendered by the needle (for acupuncture) is to drain off the noxious influences, thus expelling the disease."

5. Wang Ping equals these to the arteries of the kidneys.

"The middle region that contains elements of the Earth is the region of the 'sunlight' within the hands.[6]

"The middle region that contains elements of man is the region of the lesser Yin within the hands.[7]

"The lower region that contains the elements of Heaven is the region of the absolute Yin within the feet.[8]

"The lower region that contains the elements of Earth is the region of the lesser Yin within the feet.[9]

"The lower region that contains the element of man is the region of the great Yin within the feet.[10]

"Thus the element of Heaven within the lower region has the liver to attend to; the element of Earth within the lower region has the kidneys to attend to; and the element of man within the lower region has to attend to the force of life of the spleen and the stomach."

The Emperor asked: "And to what do the middle regions have to attend?"

Ch'i Po answered: "They too contain Heaven, they too contain Earth, and they too contain man. The element of Heaven attends to the lungs, the element of the Earth attends to the breath within the breast, and the element of man attends to the heart."

The Emperor asked: "And to what do the upper regions have to attend?"

Ch'i Po answered: "They too contain Heaven, they too contain Earth, and they too contain man. The element of Heaven attends to the corners (temples) of the head and the brows; the element of Earth attends to the corners of the mouth and the teeth; and the element of man attends to the corners of the ears and the eyes.

"Each of these three regions contains an element of Heaven, an element of Earth, and an element of man. Three elements are needed to make Heaven perfect, three elements are needed to make Earth perfect, and three elements are needed to make man perfect. The total of these three times three makes nine, and this number nine can be distinguished as the nine wild regions of the Earth; and these

6. Wang Ping equals these to the arteries of the spleen.
7. Wang Ping equals these to the arteries of the lungs.
8. Wang Ping equals these to the arteries of the lower intestines.
9. Wang Ping equals these to the arteries of the heart.
10. Wang Ping equals these to the arteries of the liver.

nine wild regions can be equaled to the nine resources (within the body).

"There are five spiritual resources[11] and there are four physical resources,[12] and taken together they amount to nine resources.

"When the five viscera cease to function they deteriorate, their color and appearance are bound to decay and death must necessarily result."

The Emperor asked: "What is the function of the subdivisions?"

Ch'i Po answered: "One must first measure those parts of the body that are fat and those that are lean, one must adjust their strength and that which is hollow and that which is solid. The solid parts must be drained while the hollow parts must be supplemented.[13]

"One must first drain blood from the arteries in order to harmonize, and then one can suppose, without further examination of the illness, that health is to be expected."

The Emperor said: "What determines life and death?"

Ch'i Po replied: "When the body is flourishing but the pulses are thin and delicate and there is little force of life, it is not in condition to resist danger.

"When the body is thin and emaciated but the pulses are large and there is too much breath within the breast, there will be death.

"When the (various) forces of the body work in mutual harmony there will be life; when they associate with each other but do not blend illness will result.

"When the three regions and the nine subdivisions mutually err[14] against each other death will result.

"When the upper and the lower, the right and the left pulses act in response to each other, as though they had gathered in order to pound grain, a great illness will ensue.

11. Wang Ping explains: The five spiritual resources are controlled by the five viscera: the liver controls the soul, or spiritual faculties (魂), the heart controls the divinely inspired part (神), the spleen controls the ideas and thoughts (意), the lungs control the inferior, or animal spirits (魄), and the kidneys control the will and resolution (志).

12. Wang Ping explains the four physical resources: 1. the temples of the head, 2. the ears and eyes, 3. the mouth and the teeth, 4. the space within the breast.

13. Wang Ping quotes: "Lao-tzu says: According to the ways of Heaven it is as injurious to have surplus as it is to be insufficiently supplied." (天 之 道 損 有 餘 補 不 足 也).

14. Wang Ping explains: 失 謂 候 不 相 來 as "are dissimilar."

"When the upper and the lower, the right and the left pulses err against each other, they cannot be calculated and death will ensue.

"When the subdivisions of the middle region are mixed together, although they should be solitary (apart from each other 獨), the viscera fail each other and death results.

"When the subdivisions of the middle region act to reduce each other death also results; and when the eye sinks (陷 = 陷) within the socket death follows."

The Emperor asked: "How can one know where the disease is located?"

Ch'i Po answered: "One investigates the nine subdivisions separately and examines separately the trifling diseases and the grave diseases, the severe ailments and the lingering (遲 = 遲 or 達, penetrating) illnesses, the diseases with fevers and the diseases with chills, and those which are accompanied by falling down.

"One takes the (pulse of the) left hand and the left foot, and then one ascends to the ankle and places one's hand about five inches above it; and one takes (the pulse of) the right hand and places one's hand upon the ankle and presses it down. When the response of the pulses can still be perceived after ascending more than five inches, and when it feels like the wriggling of a worm, there is nevertheless no disease.[15]

"When the pulses record a disturbance and feel chaotic and turbid within the hands, then there is disease. When the pulses within the hands are slow and leisurely there is also disease.

"When the pulses record that upwards they cannot reach five inches and when, after being pressed down, they do not record at all, it means death.[16] Hence when the patient loses flesh, his body can no longer walk and he must die.

"When the emanations of the middle region are suddenly interrupted (疎) or suddenly accelerated death results.

"When the pulse beats are irregular and like a hammer the disease is located within the [blood] vessels (絡 脉).

"The nine subdivisions must respond to each other. The upper ones and lower ones must work as though they were one; they must not fail each other.

15. Wang Ping adds: "the emanations are in harmony."
16. Wang Ping adds: "the emanations are interrupted and therefore the pulse can no longer respond."

"When one subdivision is in arrears, sickness follows; when two subdivisions are lagging behind, the disease that follows is grave; when three subdivisions are in arrears the disease that follows is dangerous. The so-called 'being in arrears, or lagging behind' means that not all of the subdivisions act as they should.

"By examination of man's intestines and his viscera one can come to know his dates of life and death. One must first know the vascular system, and then one can know the diseases that befall the vessels. By keeping the pulses of the viscera under supervision one is able to overcome death.

"The feet are within the region of the great Yang (太 陽). When the emanations are interrupted within the foot, the patient cannot bend down, he loses his elasticity and will die; he must wear something over his eyes (戴 眼)."

The Emperor said: "In Winter it is Yin, the female principle of darkness and death, in Summer it is Yang, the male principle of light and life—what can one say about their functions?"[17]

Ch'i Po answered: "All those pulses of the nine subdivisions that beat deeply and thinly, that are suspended and interrupted, are caused by Yin, the principle of darkness, which rules over Winter. Hence a number of deaths occur at midnight.

"All those pulse beats that are abundant, hasty, panting, and accelerated are caused by Yang, the principle of light, which rules over Summer. Hence a number of deaths occur at noon.

"For these reasons diseases brought about by heat and cold finally find their death at dawn or early morning. Those who burn within from a disease caused by heat find their death at noon.[18] Those who suffer from a disease that is caused by the wind die at the time of dusk. Those who suffer from a disease caused by water find their death at midnight. Those whose pulse beats are suddenly interrupted, or suddenly accelerated or suddenly retarded, or of sudden haste and urgency, find their death during the four seasons at the time when the sun rises.

"When the body and the flesh are worn out and fail, although the nine subdivisions still function harmoniously, there is (yet) death.

"When after seven examinations (七 診) it becomes evident that the nine subdivisions are all in accord, there will be no death. Those

17. Wang Ping adds: "Explain the time of life and death."
18. Wang Ping adds: "When Yang is at its highest."

who are described as not soon to die suffer from a disease caused by (external) influences and the menses (月 經), similar to the diseases which require seven examinations but not quite the same; and therefore the patient will not die, just as though he had the disease that required the seven examinations. But when the pulses and subdivisions become affected and ruined then the patient will die. Under these conditions he will be forced to emit retching and belching. And one must examine and question into the beginning of the illness and into its present state and location.

"Then every pulse is felt as to its urgency and compliance and the arteries (veins) and *lo* vessels are inspected as to their superficiality and depth. The upper and the lower (parts of the body) are examined as to their disorder and order. And when the pulse (脉) is in order, their illness is not a serious disease.[19] But when the pulse is tardy there is a serious disease.[20] When the pulse beats do not alternate in their coming and going death results.[21] When the disease becomes evident by the appearance of the skin death follows."[22]

The Emperor asked: "How can one treat and effect a cure?"

Ch'i Po answered: "For diseases of the arteries (經) one treats the arteries. For diseases of the capillaries (孫) and the veins one treats the capillaries and the veins and the blood, one pierces and removes. For diseases of the blood the body must have movement and one treats the arteries and the veins. When the disease is located within the weird and uncanny [substance] (奇 邪), the vessels that house the weird and uncanny must be strangled and pierced. When the patient is being retarded by being emaciated and cannot move his limbs, he must be treated with acupuncture.

"When the (pulses that indicate the state of the) upper part of the body are solid and full and those of the lower part are empty and hollow, the body is unequal in its compliance; one must search for a coagulation within the veins so that the blood can enter and the circulation can become apparent.[23]

"The pupil of the eye is the most treasured of (man's possession).

19. Wang Ping explains: "Their breath of life is strong and abundant."
20. Wang Ping adds: "Their breath of life is insufficient."
21. Wang Ping explains: "The essence and the spirit have left the body."
22. Wang Ping adds: "Then the bones are dried up and withered."
23. Wang Ping explains: "The coagulation means the coagulation of blood within the veins. This blood must be removed; then there is circulation within the tunnel of the vessels."

When the great Yang is not sufficient man must wear something over his eyes.   The sun's end or its sudden interruption casts the decision.

"Thus the requirements of life and death cannot remain undiscovered.[24]   From the fingers to the back of the hands and from the ankle upwards the breath of five fingers one must insert the needle."

24. 死生之要不可不察.

Book 7

21. *Treatise on How to Distinguish the Vascular System*

THE Yellow Emperor said: "Man's place of residence, his motion and rest (his circumstances of life), his courage and cowardice—do they not also cause change within the vascular system (pulse)?"

Ch'i Po answered: "Yes, in general man's fear and apprehension, his passion (anger) and his suffering, his motion and his rest, they all cause changes.

"Those who are about at night have difficulties in breathing emanating from the kidneys. Those whose demeanor is dissolute and licentious get a disease of the lungs. Those who are lazy and full of apprehension and fear have difficulties in breathing, emanating from the lungs. Those whose deportment is licentious and excessive will injure their spleen. Those who are full of fear and apprehension have difficulties in breathing, emanating from the lungs. Those whose demeanor is immoral and dissolute will injure their hearts.

"One should measure the degree of moisture that makes men slip and fall prostrate (度 水 跌 什[1]); they have difficulties in breathing, emanating from the kidneys and the bones.[2] At the same time those who act bravely and courageously will bring (the disease) to an end, while those who are afraid and cowardly (become infected and) fall ill.

"Therefore it is said: In order to examine the course of a disease one must investigate whether man is courageous or nervous and cowardly, and one must examine his bones, flesh, and skin and then one can know the facts of the case which are necessary for the methods of treatment.

"After heavy eating and drinking perspiration is produced by the stomach. When man is shocked and startled he does violence to his spirit and vitality, and perspiration is produced by the heart.

1. 什 = 仆.
2. Wang Ping explains: "The moist vapors penetrate the kidneys and the bones and are controlled by the kidneys."

When man carries a heavy burden while taking a long journey, perspiration is produced by the kidneys. When man, during rapid marching, is apprehensive and full of fear, perspiration is produced by the liver. When the body is shaken in hard toil perspiration is produced by the spleen.

"Thus in Spring and in Fall, in Winter and in Summer, during the four seasons and during the periods of Yin and Yang, diseases are created, that are caused by faulty practices and transgressions which have become habit.

"Food enters the stomach; its essence is then distributed into the liver and its vital force flows over into the muscles.[3]

"Food enters the stomach; its putrid gases are sent up to the heart and its essence overflows into the pulse.[4]

"The force of the pulse flows into the arteries (經) and the force of the arteries ascends into the lungs; the lungs send it into all the pulses (百 脉), which then transport its essence to the skin and the body hair. The entire vascular system unites with the secretions and passes the force of life on to a storehouse,[5] which stores the energy and vitality and intelligence. These are then transmitted to the four (parts of the body),[6] and the vital forces of the viscera are restored to their order.

"Health means restoration to order; the general expression and the perfection of the 'inch' pulse serve to decide over life and death.

"Drink enters the stomach, flows and overflows into the secretions, its essence ascends and is introduced into the spleen. The spleen distributes its secretions, which rise and enter the lungs and circulate through them. Then the general nature of liquid makes it descend and it is introduced into the bladder.

"The liquid secretions are spread in four (directions) and united in the five passages (arteries 經). This conforms to the system

3. Wang Ping explains: "The liver nourishes the muscles; thus the stomach distributes the essence of grain which enters the liver and is then absorbed and nourishes the muscles and veins."

4. Wang Ping explains: " 濁 氣 The putrid gas is that of the grain; the heart is located above the stomach. Thus the vapors of the grain enter the heart; the overflow forms a delicate essence that enters the pulse; thus the heart controls the pulse in every way."

5. Wang Ping explains: " 府 , the store-house is located where the vital forces meet; it is, in other words, the accumulation of breath that is between the two nipples and the name of it is: 'within the middle of the thorax.'"

6. Wang Ping explains those to be the upper, the lower, the internal and the external parts.

of the four seasons and the five viscera and the scheme of Yin and Yang that are held to be constant and immutable.

"When the viscera that are influenced by the great Yang alone achieve the utmost, there will be hiccoughing and laboured breathing.[7] The breath will be insubstantial and out of order, and then there is an insufficiency of Yin and a surplus of Yang. The appropriate organs outside and inside will expel that and get it out (of the body).[8]

"When the viscera that are influenced by the 'sunlight' alone achieve the utmost, there is a superabundance of the element of Yang. Then one must try to dispel some of this element of Yang and supply some of Yin which can be obtained.

"When the viscera that are influenced by the lesser Yang alone achieve the utmost, there will be convulsions;[9] the patient throws his feet forward and dies suddenly on account of that which is secreted below.[10] When the viscera that are influenced by the lesser Yang alone achieve the utmost, it means that this particular element of Yang has committed severe transgressions.

"When the viscera that are influenced by the great Yin strike out and attack, one should give it thorough attention. When the force of the five pulses (of the viscera) is reduced and the force of the stomach is not in balance, this is because of the third element of Yin.[11] A fitting treatment is to induce secretions below, that is, to supplement Yang and to drain Yin.

"When one element of Yang alone (influences the viscera), there is a whistling and hissing tone like the hiccoughs,[12] produced by the lesser Yang. Yang also strives with the upper (parts of the body) and the four pulses and seeks to dominate, and then the force of life reverts to the kidneys. A fitting treatment is then to drain the arteries (經) and the veins (*lo* vessels 絡) which are influenced by Yang, and to supplement those which are influenced by Yin.

"That which has to be achieved in regard to the first element of Yin is to treat the 'absolute Yin.' When the true (viscera) are hol-

7. 厥 here translated as 欬 to hiccough.
8. Wang Ping explains them to be the kidney and the bladder.
9. 厥氣 translated as 氣欬, convulsions.
10. 俞 translated as 輸.
11. Wang Ping explains it to be the great Yin.
12. 厥 translated as 欬.

low and insubstantial, the heart suffers from contusion,[13] the breath becomes stagnant and dense and white perspiration is produced. In order to cure the trouble one should bring about a drainage in the lower part of the body and one must blend the food with the medicines."

The Emperor asked: "What appearance have the viscera that are influenced by the great Yang?"

Ch'i Po answered: "They resemble the third element of Yang, and are given to excess and abundance."

The Emperor asked: "And what is the appearance of those viscera that are influenced by the lesser Yang?"

Ch'i Po answered: "They resemble the first element of Yang. The viscera that belong to the first element of Yang are smooth and slippery (滑) and not full and solid (實)."

The Emperor asked: "And what is the appearance of those viscera that are influenced by the 'sunlight'?"

Ch'i Po answered: "They have the appearance of abundance and superficiality. When the viscera that are under the influence of the great Yin are stricken, it means that there are hidden swellings (伏 鼓); when those under the second element of Yin are stricken, then the kidneys perish and are not light and floating."[14]

13. 肖 痛 contusions? Or like 脊 which according to K'ang-hsi tzu-tien is 痠 = muscular pains.

14. 賢 沈 不 浮 也

22. *Treatise on the Seasons as Patterns of the Viscera*

The Yellow Emperor said: "In order to bring into harmony the human body one takes as standard the laws of the four seasons and the five elements. This method serves as a regulator to man, [no matter] whether he is obedient or whether he is in opposition (to these laws), whether he is successful or whether he suffers failure. I desire further enlightenment in this matter."

Ch'i Po replied: "The five elements are metal, wood, water, fire, and earth. Their changes, their increasing value, their increasing depreciation and worthlessness serve to give knowledge of death and life and they serve to determine success and failure. They determine the strength of the five viscera, and establish their important division according to the four seasons and their dates of life and death."

The Emperor said: "I desire complete information about all this."

Ch'i Po answered: "The liver rules over Spring. The [region of the] 'absolute Yin' and the lesser Yang within the foot control the treatment and cure.[1] The days of Spring are those of the celestial stems *chia i*. When the liver suffers from an acute attack one should quickly eat sweet (food) in order to calm it down.[2]

"The heart rules over the Summer. The [region of the] lesser Yin and the region of the great Yang control the treatment and cure.[3] The days of Summer are those of the celestial stems *ping ting*. When the heart suffers from tardiness, one should quickly eat sour (food) which has an astringent effect.[4]

"The spleen rules over the long Summer.[5] The regions of the great Yin and the [regions of] 'sunlight' within the foot control the treatment and the cure.[6] The days of the long Summer are those of the celestial stems *wu chi*. When the spleen suffers from moisture one should quickly eat bitter food which has a drying effect.

"The lungs rule over Fall. The [region of the] great Yin and the region of 'sunlight' within the hands control the treatment and cure.[7] The days of Fall are those of the celestial stems *kêng hsin*. When the lungs suffer from the obstruction of the upper respiratory

1. Wang Ping explains: "The region of the 'absolute Yin' includes the pulse of the liver; the region of the lesser Yang includes the pulse of the gall bladder. The liver and the gall bladder are closely connected; hence they must be treated together."
2. Wang Ping explains: "The nature of sweet flavor is harmonizing and leisurely." Then he quotes from 全 元 起 : "When the liver suffers from an acute attack it indicates that there is an excessive fullness of the liver."
3. Wang Ping explains: "The region of the lesser Yin includes the pulse of the heart; the region of the great Yang includes the pulse of the small intestines. The heart and the small intestines are closely connected; hence they must be treated together."
4. Wang Ping explains: "The disposition of the sour flavor is to be astringent." Then he quotes from 全 元 起 : "The heart suffering from slowness means that it is devoid of strength."
5. Wang Ping explains 長 夏 to be the sixth month of the year, or its middle.
6. Wang Ping explains: "The region of the great Yin includes the pulse of the spleen, and the region of the 'sunlight' includes the pulse of the stomach. The spleen and the stomach are closely connected; hence they must be treated together."
7. Wang Ping explains: "The region of the great Yin includes the pulse of the lungs, the region of the 'sunlight' includes the pulse of the lower intestines. The lungs and the lower intestines are closely connected; hence they must be treated together."

tract, one should quickly eat bitter (food) which will disperse the obstruction and restore the flow.[8]

"The kidneys rule over Winter. The [region of the] lesser Yin and the region of the great Yang control the treatment and cure.[9] The days of Winter are those of the celestial stems *jên kuei*. When the kidneys suffer from dryness, one should quickly eat pungent food which will moisten them. It will open the pores and will bring about a free circulation of the saliva and the fluid secretions.

"Disease of the liver should be healed in Summer. When it is not healed in Summer it will become graver in Fall; when death does not strike in Fall it can be warded off in Winter. But (the disease) will arise again in Spring and then one should strictly avoid exposure to the winds.[10]

"Those who suffer from diseases of the liver should be cured during the period of the celestial stems *ping ting*.[11] When the improvement has not taken place during the period of *ping ting*, it will be the same during the period of the celestial stems *kêng hsin*.[12] When then death does not strike during the period of *kêng hsin*, it can be warded off during the period of the celestial stems *jên kuei*[13]. But the disease arises again during the period of *chia i*.[14]

"Those who have a disease of the liver are animated and quick-witted in the early morning. Their spirits are heightened in the evening and at midnight they are calm and quiet. When the liver (is sick) it has the tendency to disintegrate. Then one should quickly eat pungent food which dispels this tendency. One uses pungent food in connection with the liver in order to supplement its function and to stop leaks, and one uses sour food in order to drain and expel.

"When the disease is located within the heart it should improve

8. Wang Ping explains: The effect of bitter flavor is to widen and to disperse, therefore it is used for the lungs. He quotes 全 元 起 : "When the upper respiratory tract of the lungs is obstructed it means a surplus of air."
9. Wang Ping explains: The region of the lesser Yin includes the pulse of the kidneys; the region of the great Yang, the sun, includes the pulse of the bladder. The kidneys and the bladder are closely connected; hence they must be treated together.
10. Wang Ping adds: "It is the force of the winds that penetrates the liver, therefore there should be strict avoidance of them in order to prevent transgression."
11. The celestial stems *ping ting* correspond to Summer.
12. The celestial stems *kêng hsin* correspond to Fall.
13. The celestial stems *jên kuei* correspond to Winter.
14. The celestial stems *chia i* correspond to Spring.

during the long Summer. If it does not improve during the long Summer, it becomes graver in Winter. If in Winter death does not follow, it can be warded off in Spring; but the disease will arise again in Summer.[15] Then one should avoid eating hot food and wearing clothes[16] that produce heat.

"Those who suffer from a disease of the heart should be cured during the period of the celestial stems *wu chi*.[17] When the improvement has not taken place during the period of *wu chi*, it will be the same in the period of *jên kuei*;[18] and when death does not strike during the period of the celestial stems *jên kuei*, it can be warded off during the period of the celestial stems *chia i*.[19] But the disease arises again during the period of the celestial stems *ping ting*.[20]

"Those who suffer from a sick heart are animated and quickwitted at noon, around midnight their spirits are heightened, and in the early morning they are peaceful and quiet. A (sick) heart has the tendency to soften and to weaken. Then one should quickly eat salty food to make the heart pliable. One uses salty food in connection with the heart in order to supplement and to strengthen it, and one uses sweet food in order to drain and to dispel.

"When the disease is located within the spleen it should improve during Fall. If it does not improve during Fall it becomes graver in Spring. If in Spring death does not follow, it can be warded off in Summer; but (the disease) will arise again in the period of the long Summer. One should avoid eating warm food and eating to repletion; one should keep off swampy land and one should not wear damp clothing.

"Those who suffer from a disease of the spleen should be cured during the period of the celestial stems *kêng hsin*.[21] If it does not improve during the period of the celestial stems *kêng hsin*, it will be the same in the period of the celestial stems *chia i*.[22] And when death does not strike during the period of *chia i*, it can be warded

15. Wang Ping adds: "This is very much like the law that refers to the liver."
16. Wang Ping explains: "Heat dries out the heart; therefore it must be strictly avoided."
17. The celestial stems *wu chi* correspond to the long Summer.
18. The celestial stems *jên kuei* correspond to Winter.
19. The celestial stems *chia i* correspond to Spring.
20. The celestial stems *ping ting* correspond to Summer.
21. The celestial stems *kêng hsin* correspond to Fall.
22. The celestial stems *chia i* correspond to Spring.

off during the period of the celestial stems *ping ting*,[23] but then the disease will arise again during the period of *wu chi*.[24]

"Those who suffer from a disease of the spleen are animated and quick-witted around sunset, their spirits are heightened around sunrise and towards evening they become quiet and calm. A (sick) spleen has the tendency to work tardily and lazily; then one should quickly eat sweet food to set it at ease. One uses bitter food to drain the spleen and one uses sweet food to supplement and to strengthen it.

"When the disease is located within the lungs it should improve during Winter. If it does not improve during Winter it will become more serious in Summer. If death does not follow in Summer, it can be warded off during the period of the long Summer evenings, but the disease will again arise in Fall. One should avoid eating and drinking cold things and one should not wear chilly clothing.

"Those who suffer from a disease of the lungs should be cured during the period of the celestial stems *jên kuei*.[25] If the disease does not improve during this period, it will be the same during the period of the celestial stems *ping ting*.[26] And when death does not follow during the period of *ping ting*, it can be warded off during the period of *wu chi*,[27] but the disease will again arise during the period of *kêng hsin*.[28]

"Those who suffer from a disease of the lungs are animated and quick-witted during evening, their spirits are heightened at noon and they are calm and peaceful at midnight. (Sick) lungs have the tendency to close and to bind; then one should quickly eat sour food in order to make them receive what is due to them. One uses sour food to supplement and to strengthen the lungs and one uses pungent food to drain them and to make them expel.

"When the disease is located within the kidneys it should improve during Spring. If it does not improve during Spring it will become more serious during the period of the long Summer evenings. If death does not follow during the period of the long Summer, it can be warded off in Fall, but the disease will arise again in Winter.

23. The celestial stems *ping ting* correspond to Summer.
24. The celestial stems *wu chi* correspond to long Summer.
25. Winter.
26. Summer.
27. Long Summer
28. Fall.

One should strictly avoid burning fires, hot food, and wearing clothing which is too warm.[29]

"Those who suffer from a disease of the kidneys should be cured during the period of the celestial stems *chia i.*[30] If the disease does not improve during the period of the celestial stems *chia i*, it will become graver during the period of *wu chi.*[31] And if death does not strike during the period of *wu chi*, it can be warded off during the period of *kêng hsin*,[32] but then the disease will arise again during the period of *jên kuei.*[33]

"Those who suffer from a disease of the kidneys are quick-witted and active at midnight, and their spirits are heightened during the entire days of the last months of Spring, Summer, Fall, and Winter, and they become calm and quiet toward sunset. (Sick) kidneys have the tendency to harden; then one should eat bitter food to strengthen them. One uses bitter food to supplement and to strengthen them and one uses salty food to drain them and to make them expel.

"Thus when evil influences visit the body they must be overcome and prevented from increasing. This must be achieved by those who are healthy and whose diseases are consequently curable. This should also be achieved by those who cannot overcome the evil spirits and who consequently become more gravely ill. It also refers to those who are healthy and can ward off the disease by themselves.

"Those who are contented and satisfied with their station in life will rise above it.

"One must first ascertain the pulses of the five viscera; then one can define the intervening time, and at last one can establish the dates of life and death.[34]

29. Wang Ping explains: It is hurtful to the kidneys to become hot and dry; therefore the above-mentioned restrictions.
30. Spring.
31. Long Summer.
32. Fall.
33. Winter.
34. Wang Ping explains: The pulses of the five viscera should have the following conditions: The pulse of the liver should sound like the tone evoked from musical strings; the pulse of the heart should sound like the blows of a hammer (continuous); the pulse of the lungs should sound superficial, like a piece of wood floating on water; the pulse of the kidneys should sound like a well-regulated regiment; and the pulse of the spleen should be tremulous and at irregular intervals.

"Sickness of the liver causes swellings below both sides of the ribs, stretching the small intestines and making people prone to have fits of anger. When the liver is deficient (empty), then the eye becomes blinded and can no longer see and the ear can no longer hear. This gives to man a tendency to be afraid as though he were about to be attacked.

"(In order to cure the liver)[35] one should select from the vascular system those vessels which are controlled by the absolute Yin and by the lesser Yang. When the breathing is obstructed, this obstruction causes headaches and deafness of the ears, loss of acute perception, and swelling of the jaw.

"Sickness of the heart causes pains within the breast extending over the branches of the ribs. It causes pains below the ribs (flanks) and upon the breast. The top of the shoulders and the spaces between the fingernails hurt, and there are pains within both arms. And the entire region extending from the ribs to the flanks is affected and full of pain.

"(In order to cure the heart) one should select from the vascular system those arteries which are controlled by the lesser Yin and the great Yang, and the blood which is contained underneath the root of the tongue. Their changes indicate the diseases. One must pierce (with acupuncture) the spot which causes the disorder in order to reach the blood which is contained therein.

"Sickness of the spleen causes the body to become thick and heavy; it conditions the muscles and the flesh to have nervous spasms during sleep; the foot loses its ability to walk, there are convulsions; and pains descend the legs. When (the spleen) is deficient (empty) the stomach remains filled, the bowels give out sounds, nourishment leaks out, and food ceases to undergo the transformation (of digestion). (In order to cure the spleen) one draws blood from the arteries that are controlled by the great Yin, by the 'sunlight' and by the lesser Yin.

"Sickness of the lungs causes laboured breathing and coughing, and the air that is in disorder penetrates the top of the shoulders and the back. Perspiration emanates from the rectum, the haunches and the lap. Thighs, heels, soles and feet all are full of pain.

"When the lungs are deficient (empty), there is a decrease

35. This was added by Wang Ping.

of breathing and a lack of ability to emit and to take in breath. The ear becomes deafened and the throat turns dry.

"(In order to cure the lungs) one should select from the vascular system those arteries of the foot which are controlled by the great Yin, those arteries upon the outside of the body that are controlled by the great Yang, and those arteries within the body that are controlled by the 'absolute Yin'; and one should draw blood from them.

"Sickness of the kidneys causes the stomach to be enlarged and the shinbone to swell and tumefy. It brings about laboured breathing and coughing, the body grows heavy, perspiration comes forth during sleep,[36] which is extremely hurtful.[37]

"When the kidneys are deficient then there are pains within the thorax and the small intestines and the lower intestines hurt. The spirit becomes easily provoked[38] and annoyed, and the thoughts devoid of joy.

"(In order to cure the kidneys) one should select from the vascular system those arteries which are controlled by the lesser Yin and the great Yang, and should draw blood from them.

"The color which corresponds to the liver is green; its proper food is sweet. Non-glutinous rice, beef meat, dates and mallows are all sweet.

"The color which corresponds to the heart is red, its proper food is sour; small peas, dog-meat, plums, and leeks are all sour.

"The color which corresponds to the lungs is white; its proper food is bitter. Wheat, mutton, almonds, (apricots 杏) and scallions are all bitter.

"The color which corresponds to the spleen is yellow; its proper food is salty. Large beans, pork, chestnuts, and coarse greens are all salty.

"The color which corresponds to the kidneys is black; their proper food is pungent. Glutinous yellow panicled millet, chicken-meat, peaches and onions are all pungent.

"The pungent flavor has a dispersing effect; the sour flavor has a

36. Wang Ping explains: "When the kidneys are sick the bones cannot be used; therefore the body grows heavy."
37. Wang Ping equals 憎風 to 深惡.
38. Wang Ping explains: 清厥意樂 to mean 神躁擾故不樂.
39. Wang Ping explains: "藥 means: metal, jade, earth, stones, grasses, wood, vegetables, fruit (berries, nuts), insects (reptiles), fish, birds, and wild animals. All these can serve to expel evil influences and help to adjust and to nourish."

gathering and binding effect; the sweet flavor has a retarding effect; the bitter flavor has a strengthening effect; and the salty flavor has a softening effect.

"The poisons and medicines[39] attack the evil influences. The five grains[40] act as nourishment; the five fruits from the trees[41] serve to augment; the five domestic animals[42] provide additional benefit; the five vegetables[43] serve to complete the nourishment. Their flavors, tastes and smells unite and conform to each other in order to supply the beneficial essence (of life).

"Each of these five flavors—pungent, sour, sweet, bitter, and salty —provides a certain advantage and benefit. Their effect is either dispersing or binding and gathering, retarding or accelerating, strengthening or softening.

"Each of the diseases of the four seasons and of the five viscera reacts to that of the five flavors to which it corresponds."

40. The five grains are: non-glutinous rice, small peas, wheat, large beans, and yellow glutinous panicled millet.
41. The five tree-fruits are: peaches, plums, apricots (almonds), chestnuts, and dates.
42. The five domestic animals are: the ox, the lamb, the pig, the dog, and the chicken.
43. The five vegetables are: mallows, coarse greens, scallions, onions, and leeks.

23. *Comprehensive Explanation of the Five Atmospheric Influences*

The five flavors enter (into the organs in the following manner): the sour flavor enters into the liver; the pungent flavor enters into the lungs; the bitter flavor enters into the heart; the salty flavor enters into the kidneys; and the sweet flavor enters into the spleen. This explains where the five flavors enter.

The diseases brought about by the five atmospheric influences (五 氣) are (as follows): The heart causes belching; the lungs cause coughing; the liver causes chattering; the spleen causes difficulties in swallowing; the kidneys cause deficiencies which in turn cause sneezing and running at the nose; the stomach causes vapors, and when these are refractory they cause belching and vomiting, which in turn cause fears. The lower intestines and the small intestines cause leakages upon the burning spaces, making them overflow below and causing water (in the system). When the bladder does not function efficiently, it causes retention of urine; when it functions without restraint, it causes copious urination. The gall bladder causes fits of anger. This explains the five diseases.

The five spirits are equal to the five essences. When they are united they cause joy to emanate from the heart; they cause pity to emanate from the lungs; they cause grief to emanate from the liver; they cause anxiety to emanate from the spleen; and they cause fears to emanate from the kidneys. This explains the unity of the five spiritual essences. When the essences are exhausted then the spirits should unite.[1]

The five evils that can befall the viscera are: heat is injurious to the heart; cold is injurious to the lungs; winds are injurious to the liver; moisture is injurious to the spleen; and excessive dryness is injurious to the kidneys. This explains the five evils (惡).

The transformations of the fluid secretions as they affect the five viscera are: in regard to the heart the secretions become perspiration;[2] in regard to the lungs the secretions become mucus;[3] in regard to the liver the secretions become tears;[4] in regard to the spleen the secretions become saliva;[5] and in regard to the kidneys the secretions become spittle.[6] This explains the five fluid secretions.

In regard to the five flavors there are the following cautions and prohibitions: the pungent flavor goes into the respiratory tract; when there is an illness in the respiratory tract one should not eat too much pungent food. The salty flavor goes into the blood; when there is a disease of the blood one should not eat too much salty food. The bitter flavor goes into the bones; when there is a disease of the bones one should not eat too much bitter food. This explains the five cautions and prohibitions of what one should not eat to excess.

The five diseases originate as follows: some diseases of the element of Yin originate in the bones; some diseases of the element of Yang originate in the blood; some diseases of the element of Yin originate in the flesh; some diseases of the element of Yang originate in Sum-

1. 盧 而 相 者 也.
2. Wang Ping explains: it leaks out through the pores of the skin.
3. Wang Ping explains: the moisture comes from the nostrils.
4. Wang Ping explains: the water flows from the eyes.
5. Wang Ping explains: it flows from the lips and the mouth.
6. Wang Ping explains: it is brought forth by the teeth.

mer; and some diseases of the element of Yin originate in Winter. This explains the origin of the five diseases.

The five harmful emanations create the following disorders: when the eight evils reside within the elements of Yang in man, then the result is wildness (狂); when the eight evils reside within the elements of Yin in man, then the result is numbness.[7] When the evils strike at Yang, they cause insanity (巔); when they strike at Yin, they cause loss of speech (瘖). When the elements of Yang enter into those of Yin, the result is peace and order; but when the elements of Yin invade those of Yang, the result is an outburst of anger and rage.[8] This explains the five disorders.

The five evils that can be perceived are: the perceiving (得) in Spring of the pulse that corresponds to Fall; the perceiving in Summer of the pulse that corresponds to Winter; the perceiving during the period of the long Summer evenings of the pulse that corresponds to Spring; the perceiving in Fall of the pulse that corresponds to Summer; and the perceiving in Winter of the pulse of the long Summer. All this means that Yin [the female principle of darkness] enters into Yang [the male principle of light and life]; consequently the disease is likely to be aggravated and cannot be cured. This explains the five (perceptible) evils. It is decreed that they all lead to death and cannot be cured.

The five viscera hide and store the following: the heart stores and harbors the divine spirit (神); the lungs harbor the animal spirits (魄); the liver harbors the soul and the spiritual faculties (魂); the spleen harbors ideas and opinions (意); and the kidneys harbor will power and ambition (志). This explains what is stored away and harbored by the five viscera.

The control of the five viscera acts in the following way: the heart controls the pulse; the lungs control the skin; the liver controls the muscles and sinews; the spleen controls the flesh; and the kidneys control the bones. This explains the five controls.

The five exertions that are hurtful to the body are: the extended

---

7. Wang Ping explains: "When the evil dwells within the pulse of the Yang element, then the four limbs are feverish and full; therefore it causes madness and wildness. When the five evils reside within the pulse of the Yin element, then the six arteries prevent the passage of liquid, there is no flow within and thus numbness results."

8. Wang Ping says: "when Yang enters into Yin the disease will quiet down; when Yin enters into Yang the disease will rise angrily (怒)."

use of the eyes hurts the blood;[9] to lie down and to rest for a long time is hurtful to the respiratory tract;[10] to be in a sitting position for too long a time is hurtful to the flesh;[11] to stand up for a long time is hurtful to the bones;[12] and to walk for a long time is hurtful to the muscles.[13] This explains the five exertions that are hurtful to the body.

The five pulses should correctly appear in the following ways: The pulse of the liver should sound like the strings of a musical instrument; the pulse of the heart should sound like the blows of a hammer (continuous); the pulse of the spleen should be intermittent and irregular; the pulse of the lungs should be (soft) like hair (and feathers);[14] the pulse of the kidneys should sound like a stone.[15] This explains the pulses of the five viscera.

9. Wang Ping explains: the exertion affects the heart.
10. Wang Ping explains: the exertion affects the lungs.
11. Wang Ping explains: the exertion affects the spleen.
12. Wang Ping explains: the exertion affects the kidneys.
13. Wang Ping explains: the exertion affects the liver.
14. The words in parentheses are Wang Ping's interpretation.
15. Wang Ping explains: It should sound deep and strong like a stone thrown.

24. The Order and Scope of Man's Vigor and Constitution

The constant order of man is that in the region of the great Yang there is always much blood and little breath; in the regions of the lesser Yang there is always little blood and much breath; in the regions of 'sunlight' there is always much breath and much blood; in the regions of the lesser Yin there is always little blood and much breath; in the regions of the 'absolute Yin' there is always much blood and little breath; and in the regions of the great Yin there is always much breath and little blood. This is the heaven-determined constant order.[1]

With regard to the foot: the great Yang and the lesser Yin act like coat and lining; the lesser Yang and the absolute Yin act like coat and lining; the 'sunlight' and the great Yin act like coat and lining. This is the relationship between Yin and Yang in regard to the foot.

1. Wang Ping explains: "There is a heaven-determined constant order for the amount of vigor and energy. Therefore one always uses the method of acupuncture to dispel and to drain off excessive (vigor)."

With regard to the hand: the great Yang and the lesser Yin act like coat and lining; the lesser Yang and the palm of the hand (心 主) act like coat and lining; the 'sunlight' and the great Yin act like coat and lining. This is the relationship between Yin and Yang in regard to the hand.

Nowadays it is known that in order to cure completely the suffering of hand and foot, of Yin and Yang, one must first remove blood; and by such means one also removes the ailment, which can then be examined; and, if desirable, one can afterwards drain off the surplus and supplement when there is an insufficiency.

In order to obtain information about the back one must first measure the space between the two breasts and calculate the proportion of change. One takes this as a rough measure. After this space is halved, one has two coves which support each other. It is then recommended to measure the back. Thus the first cove is in the upper part of the body. Along the ridge of the spinal column there are two coves in the lower part of the body. It is in these lower coves that the lungs should be located. If one repeats this measure further down one finds the heart. One measure farther below in the left corner one finds the liver, and in the right corner there is the spleen; and one measure further down there are the kidneys. This explains the measures (and locations) of the five viscera for the purpose of applying moxa treatment and piercing (for acupuncture).

When the body is content but will and ambition are in distress, disease arises from the pulse; and in order to cure it one uses moxa treatment and acupuncture.

When the body is content and full of pleasure, and when ambition is gratified and happy, then disease arises from the flesh;[2] and in order to cure it one uses acupuncture.

When the body is in distress but the will and ambition are gratified and happy, disease arises from the muscles; and in order to cure it one uses moxa (irons? 熨) and breathing exercises.[3]

When the body is afflicted and will and ambition are also in distres, disease arises from the (difficulties of the) throat in swallowing and gulping. In order to cure this, one applies every kind of medicine.

2. Wang Ping explains: Then bones and muscles do no longer exert themselves.
3. Wang Ping explains 熨 引 to mean 藥 熨 導 引.

When the body is frequently startled and frightened, the circulation in the arteries and the veins ceases, and disease arises from numbness and the lack of sensation. In order to cure this, one uses massage and medicines prepared from the lees of wine. This explains the five (conditions) of the body and the will.

When one punctures the region of the 'sunlight', blood and air are issued forth; when one punctures the region of the great Yang, blood and noxious air are issued forth; when one punctures the region of the lesser Yang, air and foul blood are issued forth; when one punctures the region of the lesser Yin, air and blood are issued forth; when one punctures the region of the absolute Yin, blood and noxious air are issued forth.

Book 8

25. *Treatise on the Value of Life and the Achievement of a Perfect Body*

THE Yellow Emperor said: "Covered by Heaven and supported by Earth,[1] all creation together in its most complete perfection is planned for the greatest achievement: Man. Man lives on the breath of Heaven and Earth and he achieves perfection through the laws of the four seasons. The ruler as well as the masses share their utmost desire: the wish for a perfect body.

"Since the circumstances and the facts of the ailments and diseases of the body are unknown, the daily excesses are continued and become profoundly manifest upon the bones, the marrow, the heart, and the private parts, which suffer and contract diseases.[2]

"I desire to know whether and how acupuncture will remove these diseases."

Ch'i Po replied: "The flavor of salt is salty; its emanations cause the organs to produce moist secretions.

"When (the pulse of the liver that sounds like) the strings of a musical instrument is interrupted, its tone becomes loud and jarred. When the wood (the element of the liver) spreads and develops it produces leaves.[3] Thus when disease penetrates deeply the noises that are connected with it are vomiting and belching.[4] Thus there are three injuries that can befall man's inner organs.[5]

"Poisons and medicines cannot cure these shortcomings, the needle cannot extract all of them; therefore one must cut the skin and wound the flesh, and the blood which is attacked by the (incoming) air is of black color."[6]

1. Compare with *Chung Yung* (中 庸), chapter 25.
2. Wang Ping quotes 太 素, which equals 慮 to 患.
3. Wang Ping explains: "When wood distributes its vigor it becomes manifest at the outside and it becomes flourishing in all its branches. Thus the disease must affect the center of the lobes of the lungs."
4. Wang Ping explains: "the lungs store unclean blood, therefore these noises."
5. The inner organs here referred to are according to Wang Ping: the liver, the lungs, the thorax. The three injuries are: when the pulse that sounds like musical strings is interrupted; when the lobes of the lungs cause a disease; and when the tones change into vomiting and belching.
6. The disease is transferred upon the interior of the lungs, therefore the poisons and medicines

The Emperor said: "I should like to keep in mind the pains and irritations: those that are deluding and cause disorder, and those that react by aggravating the disease. We cannot change them and substitute others and therefore should we not make them known to the people so that they can consider them as injurious and destructive?"

Ch'i Po answered: "Man draws life from Earth, but his fate depends upon Heaven. Heaven and Earth unite to bestow life-giving vigor as well as destiny upon man.[7]

"Man has the ability to conform to the four seasons. Heaven and Earth act as his father and mother. He who is aware of the (needs) of all human beings is called the Son of Heaven (天 子).[8]

"For Heaven there exists Yin [the female element of darkness] and Yang [the male element of light]; for man there are the twelve divisions of time. Heaven has cold and heat; man has (the abstract and the concrete,) the hollow and the solid.

"One can take as invariable rule: Heaven and Earth; the changes between Yin and Yang; the infallibility of the four seasons; the knowledge of the methods of the twelve divisions of time.[9] Not even imperial wisdom can take advantage of these or oppress them.[10]

"Imperial wisdom can preserve the changes of the eight winds,[11] and the changes of mutual destruction which have been established for the five elements.[12] Imperial power can apprehend the fate of that which is deficient and that which is substantial and full, the fate of those who walk away alone and those who enter alone, those who yawn and those who sigh, and imperial wisdom must become aware of the tiniest and most trifling circumstances."

---

cannot cure it. The arteries and the veins are not at the exterior, consequently the needle is too short and cannot extract all the disease. Therefore the skin must be cut and the flesh must be injured, and only then can one attack the foul blood which has been in the lungs for too long a time. The air can then again communicate and strike. The blood which becomes then visible is of black color. (Wang Ping's commentary).

7. 天 地 合 氣 命 之 曰 人.

8. Wang Ping adds: "He who is aware of the origin of all living beings and of Heaven and Earth as unfailing providers is called the Son of Heaven."

9. Wang Ping explains: The twelve divisions, in regard to the exterior, refer to the atmospheric divisions which must be the twelve months. In regard to the interior it represents the twelve pairs of main vessels.

10. 聖 智 不 能 欺 也.

11. Wang Ping explains: 八 動 to mean 八 節 風 變 動.

12. Wang Ping explains: 五 勝 to mean 五 行 之 氣 相 勝.

The Emperor said: "While man is alive he has a body, a physical shape, from which he cannot part. Yin and Yang, Heaven and Earth combine their life-giving emanations; a part of these are the nine uncultivated regions of the earth, and a part are the four seasons and the seasons and the months, of which there are big and small ones; the days, of which there are short and long ones, and all in creation that lives—and all these can by no means overcome their limitations and measures. Thus I dare to ask you to give to me the formula of what to do about that which is deficient and that which is substantial and solid, and about those who yawn and those who sigh."

Ch'i Po explained: "When the element of wood reaches the element of metal it is felled; when the element of fire reaches the element of water it will be extinguished; when the element of the earth is reached by the element of wood it is penetrated; when the element of metal reaches the element of fire it is dissolved; and when water reaches the earth its flow is interrupted and cut off. Although the living creatures are the utmost (in perfection), they cannot overcome exhaustion.

"The method of the needle (acupuncture) is available to all the people; but the people know only how to live, they do not understand how to apply the five methods in order to get well from their diseases. The first method cures the spirit; the second gives knowledge of how to nourish the body; the third gives knowledge of the true effects of poisons and medicines; the fourth explains acupuncture and the use of the small and the large needle; the fifth tells how to examine and to treat the intestines and the viscera, the blood and the breath. These five methods are drawn up together so that each has one that precedes it.

"Nowadays, in this latest period, acupuncture is applied in order to supply what is lacking and in order to drain off excessive fullness. All those who work (in these fields) share this knowledge.

"Since these methods are those of Heaven, the Earth follows and adjusts its action. Those who are in harmony are like an echo; those who are in accord with these methods are like shadows; they follow (their way) Tao, and need neither demons nor gods, for they are free and independent."

The Emperor said: "I desire to hear about their way!"

Ch'i Po replied: "In order to make all acupuncture thorough and

effective one must first cure the spirit. Then after one has established (the pulse) of the five viscera and determined the nine sub-
divisions（九 候）, one can apply the needle.

"All the pulses remain invisible and one should disregard all
dangerous appearances; but one should rely upon one's combined
examinations of the external and the internal circumstances, and one
should not rely upon past experience. If one toys with the appearance and disappearance (of diseases), they will be transferred
upon man.

"Man has five deficiencies and five solid parts. Even when the
deficiencies are not close (to the eye) and even when the solid and
healthy parts are not far away, it is difficult to distinguish (瞋? = 瞬)
between the apparent manifestations of the state of health.

"The action of the hand is of utmost importance; then the performance of the needle is splendid and uniform.[13] Mere silent
meditation, the observation of the right conduct and the beholding
of pleasurable sights and their changes are called groping in the dark,
and the resulting confusion does not reveal the form of the disease.[14]

"If one watches a crow while the crow discovers some paniceled
millet, it flies rapidly in compliance with its discovery—would its
(action) be unconscious and without sensibility? It lies in ambush
like the horizontal parts of a crossbow, and it rises as though it were
set forth by the moving power (of the universe)."

The Emperor asked: "What can be done about deficiencies（虛）
and about the solid and substantial parts（實）?"

Ch'i Po answered: "When one applies acupuncture to the defi-
ciencies（虛）one will necessarily supplement them; and when one
punctures the substantial parts (the excessive fullness) one will
necessarily drain them. When the vigor of the arteries has come
to an end, one should attend to them with great care so that they
do not fail completely. Those who concentrate their minds upon
the depth or the superficiality (of the disease) treat distance and
nearness as though it were the same. Those who are at the point
of an abyss feel as though their hands were in the grip of a tiger;

13. Wang Ping explains: "then the body is bright and clean, and there is uniformity and health
in its upper and lower parts."
14. 靜 意 視 義 觀 適 之 變 謂 冥 冥 莫 知 其 形

at that time their energy and care are not devoted to the care of all creation."[15]

15. 神 無 營 扵 衆 物 .

Wang Ping explains: "Those who have in mind depth and superficiality know whether the disease is external or internal. Those who treat distance and nearness as though it were the same make a distinction between depth and superficiality. Those who are at the point of an abyss cannot dare to be careless, and those whose hands are in the grip of a tiger yearn to be strong. If the energy and the spirit are not directed to care for all creatures, if the spirit is not peaceful and the diseases under supervision, man should look neither to the left nor to the right."

26. *Treatise on the Eight Principal Divine Manifestations*

The Yellow Emperor asked: "In order to make use of the services of the needle one must follow certain laws (法) and methods (則). What is the nature of these laws and methods nowadays?"

Ch'i Po answered: "The laws are those of Heaven, and the methods are those of Earth; in order to combine them one follows (the system of) the heavenly lights."

The Emperor said: "I should like to have complete information about this."

Ch'i Po explained: "All the laws of acupuncture must attend upon the sun, the moon, the planets, the stars, and the four seasons. These are the eight factors of the atmosphere, and when the atmosphere is established one can apply acupuncture.

"Thus when the weather is warm and the sun clear and bright, the blood of man flows gently and his secretions protect his breath (vigor) and keep it volatile. Hence the blood flows easily and the breath moves smoothly.

"When the weather is cold and the sun is darkened, man's blood coagulates and does not flow,[1] and his hitherto protected breath sinks low and perishes.

"When the moon begins to wax, then blood and breath come to life, the essences receive new incentive and guard the breath of life which begins to be active. When the moon is full to the rim, there is abundance of blood and breath (within man), the muscles and the flesh are firm and strong. When the moon is empty to the rim, the muscles and the flesh become reduced, the arteries and the

1. Dictionary of K'ang Hsi explains 泣 to mean 血 凝 不 消 .

veins become empty, and the hitherto guarded breath departs, leaving the body in a deserted (solitary) condition. Therefore one should act in accordance with the weather and the seasons in order to have blood and breath thoroughly adjusted and harmonized— and consequently—when the weather is cold, one should not apply acupuncture.[2] But when the day is warm there should not be any hesitation about (the advisability of acupuncture).[3]

"At the time of the new moon one should not drain, and when the moon is full one should not supplement. When the moon is empty to the rim one can not heal diseases; hence one should consult the weather and the seasons and adjust (the treatment) to them. According to the order of Heaven the periods of abundance and want influence the (heavenly) lights; they assign the positions of the lights and regulate them, and therefore one should attend (to these periods).

"Hence when the sun and the moon are still new and one applies draining, the result is deficiency of the viscera.[4] When the moon is full and one supplements the blood and the vigor, they will spread and overflow; within the veins there will be a stoppage of blood, and they are then called heavily filled (overloaded).

"To undertake a cure when the moon is empty to the rim means disorder and confusion of the regular conduct; Yin and Yang will conflict with each other (within the body), and that which is right and correct and that which is evil and harmful cannot be distinguished. Deterioration has set in, there is deficiency at the outside and disorder and confusion in (the body), and excess and evil will arise."

The Emperor asked: "Why must the planets, the stars, and the temperature of the eight principal factors (八 正) be taken into consideration?"

Ch'i Po replied: "The planets and the stars (must be considered) because they determine the course of sun and moon;[5] the atmosphere of the eight principal factors (must be considered) because they attend to the deficiencies and harmful emanations of the eight winds, and, ultimately, the seasons. Among the four seasons one can dis-

2. Wang Ping adds: "For then the blood congeals and ceases to flow and the hitherto guarded breath perishes."
3. Wang Ping adds: "For then the blood flows gently and the breath (vigor) moves smoothly."
4. Wang Ping explains: "blood and breath weaken."
5. 星 辰 所 以 制 日 月 之 行 .

tinguish between Spring, Autumn, Winter, and Summer; and the breath of each season has its particular place and it takes (all) the seasons to harmonize the breath.[6] By means of the regular temperature of the eight principal factors one can avoid the deficiencies and the harmful emanations and one can avoid violations.[7]

"When the weakness of the body coincides with the deficiency of the breath, the two deficiencies mislead each other and their force enters the bones and in turn inflicts hurt upon the five viscera.

"But if those who are experts in medical treatment take into consideration the time of the treatment they will not inflict any hurt. There it is said: Those who do not fear certain kinds of atmosphere are ignorant."[8]

The Emperor said: "How excellent is this method of following the stars and the planets which I have just heard! But I am also desirous of hearing about the methods of the past."

Ch'i Po replied: "Within the methods of the past there was a fore-knowledge of the needle (of acupuncture) applied to the arteries; their examinations came down to the present day: there was a fore-knowledge of the fact that the days were cold and warm, that the moon was vacant and full and that one should take into consideration the lightness and the heaviness of the atmosphere and the effect of their blending in regard to the body. By observation of these arrangements one derives verification. To examine into that which is deep and profound means (to examine) the body and the breath, but the blood and the vital essences are not apparent upon the outside of the body. Only those who are experts in the art of examination have the knowledge (of decay and prosperity of the body).[9]

"They take into consideration whether the day is cold or warm, whether the moon is empty or full, they consider the four seasons and whether the atmosphere is light or heavy; and they consider how these factors associate with each other, their mutual affinity and their blending and harmony.

6. Wang Ping explains: "the location for the breath of the four seasons can be defined: the breath of Spring is within the arteries and the pulse, the breath of Summer lies within the capillaries and the veins, the breath of Fall lies within the skin, and the breath of Winter lies within the bones and the marrow."

7. Wang Ping adds: "and then there will be no sickness."

8. Wang Ping explains: "The atmosphere that should be avoided is harmful and brings diseases; thus those who cannot avoid it are ignorant."

9. The words in parentheses were added by Wang Ping.

"The physician must always observe these things first, notwithstanding the lack of symptoms upon the outside (of the body). Therefore it is said: one should inquire into and examine that which is profound and mysterious. Perpetrated ad infinitum these methods can be transmitted to posterity, and this explains the extraordinary ways of the physician.[10] Because of the fact that symptoms cannot be perceived upon the outside not everybody can see them.[11]

"About those who are able to see without need for symptoms and who are able to taste when there are no flavors—it is said that they make use of profound and mysterious (knowledge) and that they resemble those who are divinely inspired.

"What does it mean to be weak and affected by evil influences? It is the atmosphere of the eight principal factors that can bring about weakness and evil influences.

"What is right and what is harmful? When the body uses all its strength, perspiration flows freely through the open pores and encounters the minute but weakening influences with man. Thus one does not know their circumstances and one is unable to see their form.

"The superior physician helps before the early budding of the disease. He must first examine the three regions of the body (三　部) and define the atmosphere of the nine subdivisions (九　候) so that they are entirely in harmony, and nothing can be destroyed, and then his help sets in. Therefore he is called the superior physician.

"The inferior physician begins to help when (the disease) has already developed; he helps when destruction has already set in. And since his help comes when the disease has already developed it is said of him that he is ignorant. The three divisions of the body and the nine subdivisions then contend with each other and the disease will therefore be destructive.

"If one knows the location of the disease, one knows through examination that the diseases of the three regions of the body and the nine subdivisions are located within the pulse, and one can thus treat and cure them. Therefore it is said that one should attend

10. Wang Ping explains: "The physician is different from the common man—those who are common and vulgar are not able to see."

11. Wang Ping explains: "These methods were made known and could thus be handed down to posterity. If posterity does not interrupt them their use must be transmitted ad infinitum. These methods alone permit one to see and to know. And this is the reason why the doctor who has studied them is different from the common man."

to the gates of the pulse. To be ignorant of these circumstances means to see evil appearances.''

The Emperor said: ''I should like to receive information about what happens when supplementing and draining do not achieve their purpose.''

Ch'i Po answered: ''In order to drain one must use *fang* (方), the right condition or method. *Fang* means that one must apply (draining) when the atmospheric condition is favorable, one must apply it when the moon is full, one must apply it when the day is warm, and one must apply it when the body is in an orderly state. One must apply it when the breath is being inhaled. Then the needle must be inserted, and it must be repeated when the breath is being inhaled again. But the needle must be turned around, and this must be repeated when the breath is being exhaled; and then the needle must be slowly drawn out.

''Therefore it is said: In order to drain one must use *fang* (方), the right condition, in regard to the breath (氣) and its procedure. In order to supplement one must use *yüan* (員), to round out. What is this rounding out? It refers to the procedure (行);[12] and this procedure means to transmit and to shift.

''In order to puncture one must enter the blood (stream) repeatedly, and one uses the moment of inhalation to push the needle. Thus *fang*, the right condition, and *yüan*, the rounding out, (tell us) when not to apply the needle. Hence, in order to nourish and care for the spirit and mind, one must be aware of the appearances of the body: whether it is fat or thin, whether the blood, the vital essences, the constitution and breath are flourishing or deteriorating. Constitution and breath determine man's spirit and energy and one should not be heedless of their nourishment and care.''[13]

The Emperor said: ''How wonderful this reasoning! To bring into agreement man's body with Yin and Yang, the two principles in nature, and with the four seasons; his echoing of want and full-

12. Wang Ping explains: ''行 means: to drain off that which is stagnant. The vigor must necessarily be drained so that one can proceed. 移 means: to shift that which does not renew itself. In order to have the pulse in a healthy condition the blood must renew itself.''
13. Wang Ping explains: ''When the spirit is calm and peaceful there will be a long life. If one neglects the spirit the body becomes injured; therefore one should not be heedless of the nourishment and care of the spirit.''

ness, his response to the most subtle influences; who but you could so interpret it? However, you distinguish and describe the body and the spirit. What is meant by *hsing*, the body [the visible form], and what is meant by *shên*, the spirit? I desire to hear it all."[14]

Ch'i Po replied: "Let me discuss *hsing*, the body [the visible form]. What is the body? The body is regarded as holding that which is subtle and minute, and it is held responsible and investigated for its diseases. By searching into it and pondering over its regular conduct (經), much will become apparent; but to place the hand in front of it does not reveal the facts (details) of the case. Therefore it is called *hsing* the body, the physical appearance."

The Emperor asked: "And what is meant by *shên* (神), the spirit?"

Ch'i Po answered: "Let me discuss *shên*, the spirit. What is the spirit? The spirit cannot be heard with the ear. The eye must be brilliant of perception and the heart must be open and attentive, and then the spirit is suddenly revealed through one's own consciousness. It cannot be expressed through the mouth; only the heart can express all that can be looked upon. If one pays close attention one may suddenly know it but one can just as suddenly lose this knowledge. But *shên*, the spirit, becomes clear to man as though the wind has blown away the cloud. Therefore one speaks of it as the spirit.

"The three sections of the body and the nine subdivisions are the original elements. The treatise on the nine needles is not enough by itself."

14. Wang Ping explains: "神 means: the spirit and the energy that can be thoroughly understood by knowledge and wisdom. 形 means: the body that can be examined in order to treat it."

27. *Treatise on the Parting and Meeting of that Which is Beneficial and that which is Harmful*

The Yellow Emperor asked: "I hear that there are nine needles and nine treatises (篇) and hence you have given these nine. But nine times nine makes eighty-one treatises and I wish to understand thoroughly the meaning of all of them.

"The invariable rule says: 'breath becomes abundant and it decreases, it is to the left and to the right, and it is changed and shifted.

That which is above blends (調) with that which is below, and that which is at the left harmonizes with that which is at the right. If there is a surplus or an insufficiency, one supplements or drains, whichever is desirable for the blood.' I am aware of all this. Here the blood and the vital substances are shifted where the deficiencies and excessive fullnesses arise, and noxious influences cannot enter from the outside into the arteries (經).

"But I desire to know: when the evil influences are within the arteries how can the disease be taken out of people?"

Ch'i Po answered: "The calculations necessarily correspond to Heaven and Earth. Thus Heaven has the rules (度) and the constellations, the Earth has (the law of) the main arteries of water, and man has the vascular system.[1]

"When Heaven and Earth are warm and gentle, then the main arteries of the water are peaceful and quiet. When Heaven is cold and the Earth is icy (frozen), then the main arteries of water are stiffened and frozen. When Heaven is very hot and the Earth is heated, the arteries of water boil over. When suddenly a fierce and scorching wind arises, the arteries of water will show high waves and flow rapidly and rise up.[2] Now evil influences can enter the pulse. When there is cold the blood congeals; when there is heat the breath comes smoothly and gently. Because of deficiency and evil, alien matter can enter (into the pulse), just as the wind can affect the arteries of water. To be constant and regular is best for the movement of the pulse. Moreover there are times when an up-surge (隴 起) affects the pulse, but then it should also be orderly and methodical.

"The 'inch' pulse extends to the center of the hand. It is sometimes large and sometimes small. When it is large then it is most harmful, when it is small then it is regular and healthy; but its procedure is not permanently adjusted.

"With reference to the elements of Yin and those of Yang one

1. Wang Ping explains: "宿 means: the twenty-eight Chinese zodiacal constellations; 度 means: the 365 measures of the year; 經 水 means: the waters of the oceans, the waters of the great rivers, the water of the lakes, the waters of the great streams, the rivers, and the brooks. Within the earth these waters form the main arteries; therefore they are called the arteries of water. The vascular system of the pulse means the pulses of the hands and the feet, the pulses of the three regions of Yin and the three regions of Yang—they are all considered as the vascular system."

2. Wang Ping adds: "Man's vascular system acts accordingly."

is not able to apply measurements. One therefore proceeds to examine the three sections of the body and the nine subdivisions for sudden occurrences and early interruptions in their course. One should insert the needle at the time of inhalation. One should not allow the breath to conflict with the needle. When the needle is inserted one should rest it there for a moment, and the breathing of the patient must be quiet. One should not allow evil influences to enter the body. While the patient is still inhaling one should give a little turn to the needle. The needle should be taken out at the time of exhalation, but it should not be taken out suddenly; and when the breath is completely exhaled one should withdraw the needle. This procedure is called 'draining.'"

The Emperor asked: "What is to be done when supplementing is insufficient?"

Ch'i Po answered: "One must first feel with the hand and trace the system of the body. One should interrupt the sufficiencies and distribute them evenly, one should apply binding and massage. One should attack the sick part and allow it to swell, one should pull it and make it subside, one should distribute it and get hold of the evil.

"On the outside one should treat the openings which are left by the needle so that they close up and so that the spirit can remain within. When all the breath is spent at the exhalation, one should insert the needle and wait for some time until the patient has to inhale, as though one waited for something precious, and were unconscious of day and night. When the breath is entirely exhausted in exhalation, one should move the needle, but with great care and caution.

"If at the time of inhalation the needle is withdrawn, the breath cannot leave the body and everything is at its proper place. (By these means) one pushes shut the gates (of the body) and causes the spirit and the breath to be kept inside. And the detention of an extensive quantity of vigor is called to 'supplement.'"

The Emperor asked: "What part is played by subdivisions and breath(候 氣 奈 何)?"

Ch'i Po answered:"The evil influences are removed from the veins (*lo* vessels 絡) and enter the arteries(經), and thence they are released into the blood within the pulse.

"When the cold and the heat (the temperature of the body) are not in mutual agreement, like the rising of the bubbling waves which sometimes come and sometimes recede, then the normal temperature of the body cannot be maintained.

"Therefore it is said: When a wave of temperature comes one must take hold of it and interrupt a sudden change of temperature and one must apply draining without obstruction of the thoroughfare. Vigorous breath means normal breath. Hence it is said: if the normal breath becomes too low, one should not obstruct the tendency of those waves that are coming up.

"Thus when one does not recognize harmful breathing one lets the normal breath pass by. If one then cures the disease by draining, the vigorous constitution becomes weakened without being supplemented; the evil will again enter the body of the patient, and the original disease will be aggravated.

"Therefore it is said: If the departure (of the evil influences) cannot be instant and final, then the disease may flare up as mentioned before.

"One cannot suspend anything by means of a hair (不 可 挂 以 髮); thus one should treat the evil until the time when it is completely exhausted and has been sent forth by means of draining. Whether early or late, the blood and the vigor are then completely freed [of the disease], which cannot descend.

"Therefore it is said: Those who know the right opportunity and the right way will not use a hair to hang up anything, but those who are ignorant of the right opportunity may wield a hammer and the disease will not come out. This is the meaning."

The Emperor asked: "When are supplementing and draining indicated?"

Ch'i Po answered: "In order to attack the evil, the disease has to become manifest so that it can be expelled.[3] Then the blood becomes flourishing and the normal temperature is restored.

"If this illness is a recent guest in the body and if it is abundant, it does not yet have a fixed abode, and in order to expel it one uses the front; and in order to draw it out one brings to a stop the refractory forces by applying acupuncture to the warm blood. When acupuncture causes the blood to appear, the disease can be established and can be terminated."

3. Wang Ping adds: "In order to examine the disease one must have (some of the patient's) blood and then one can get hold of the illness."

The Emperor said: "Excellent! However, when the normal and evil exist side by side, does not then the breath (temperature) rise up in waves?"

Ch'i Po answered: "One examines by feeling with the hand the three sections of the body and the nine subdivisions, as to whether they are overly abundant or wanting, and one brings them into harmony.[4]

"One examines the patient's left side, then his right side, the upper and lower parts of his body for any visible fault, or any visible reduction. In order to examine disease of the viscera one determines (their breath and applies acupuncture).[5]

"Not to know the three sections of the body means not to discriminate between Yin and Yang, and not to distinguish between Heaven and Earth. The Earth has the climate of the Earth, and Heaven has the climate of Heaven. Man harmonizes these (climates) within his bowels by means of the fixed pattern of the three regions of his body.

"Therefore it is said: The physician who applies acupuncture without knowing about the three regions of the body and the nine subdivisions, even when the disease is located within the pulse, nevertheless commits a grave error which will reach its extreme, since the physician cannot be forbidden to practice.

"If (for instance) an emperor punished his people although they had not committed any transgressions, this would be called a great fault. (One can apply this to medicine:[6]) if a physician reverses and spoils the natural condition of a body, health can never again be recovered. Those who use fullness in order to create emptiness, those who use evil in order to bring about normalcy, and those who use the needle without the right way, those physicians will only bring about a contrary (wrong) reaction and hurt the patient's normal health. Instead of bringing about compliance they bring about resistance. Blood and vital substances become scattered and spoiled, the normal constitution becomes completely lost and evil influences alone reign inside the body. This interrupts

---

4. Wang Ping explains: "Overabundance(盛)indicates draining; want (虛) indicates supplementing. If the patient is neither overabundant nor wanting he is normal. In order to take hold of the disease one follows this rule."
5. The words in parentheses were added by Wang Ping.
6. The words in parentheses were added by Wang Ping.

man's long life and brings disaster over the patient.   Finally, those who do not know the three regions of the body and the nine sub-divisions will not be able to practice medicine for long.

"Therefore, not to know and to combine the four seasons and the five elements increases their fighting among each other; this frees the evil forces and assaults the normal condition, thus cutting short man's (the patient's) long life.

"When the evil is a recent guest in the body it does not yet have a fixed abode and can be expelled.   In order to do so it is brought forward where it can be met and detained.   And then, by means of draining, the disease is brought to an immediate end."

28. *A Thorough Discussion of the Hollow and the Solid, The Fullness and the Insufficiency (of the Body)*

The Yellow Emperor asked: "What is meant by emptiness and fullness?"

Ch'i Po answered: "When harmful influences are plentiful then we can speak of fullness; when the essences are decreased we can speak of emptiness."[1]

The Emperor asked: "What can be done about emptiness and fullness?"[2]

Ch'i Po answered: "When the breath is wanting, the lungs are empty; when the breath is refractory, the feet are cold.   If this does not happen at the same time, then the patient will live.[3]   If it does happen at the same time, the patient will die.   The rest of the viscera all act accordingly and alike."

The Emperor asked: "What is meant by doubly full (重 實)?"

Ch'i Po answered: "The so-called double fullness (or state of repletion) is described as great fevers, hot vapors, and a full pulse— all these phenomena are called double fullness."

The Emperor asked: "When the arteries and the veins are all too full, what can one do about them?   Can they be treated and cured?"

Ch'i Po answered: "When the arteries (經) and the veins (絡) are full, then the 'inch' pulse becomes accelerated and hasty and the

---

1. Wang Ping explains: "奪 means: the essences decrease and are reduced as though they were snatched away."

2. Wang Ping adds: "This means the principle of the emptiness and fullness of the five viscera."

3. 非 其 時 則 生 當 其 時 則 死.

'cubit' pulse becomes retarded.   All this should be treated.   Therefore it is said: (when the pulse is) smooth then it is in compliance,
when it is rough (澀) and uneven then it is in disorder.   Hence
fullness and emptiness (strength and weakness) should be distributed
in compliance with the original form of each category; then the five
viscera, the bones, and the flesh work smoothly (produce a smooth
pulse) and with profit and will last for a long time."

The Emperor asked: "What can be done when the vigor of the
veins is insufficient and the vigor of the arteries is in surplus?"

Ch'i Po answered: "What does happen when the vigor of the veins
(*lo* vessels) is insufficient and the vigor of the arteries is in surplus?
Then the mouth of the pulse is hot (feverish), while the 'cubit' pulse
is cold (chills).   Autumn and Winter bring about disorder, while in
Spring and Summer there is order.   All this influences and controls
the diseases."[4]

The Emperor said: "What can be done when the arteries are
empty and the veins are full?"

Ch'i Po answered: "When the arteries are empty and the veins
are full, the 'cubit' pulse is hot and full and the mouth of the pulse
is cold and rough.   Then death will occur during the Spring and
Summer, and life will continue during Fall and Winter."

The Emperor asked: "How can one treat all this?"

Ch'i Po answered: "When the veins are full and the arteries are
empty, one applies cauterization by burning moxa at (the regions of)
Yin and one applies the needle of acupuncture to (the regions of)
Yang.   When the arteries are full and the veins are empty, then
one applies the needle of acupuncture to (the regions of) Yin and
cauterizes by burning moxa at (the regions of) Yang."

The Emperor asked: "What is meant by doubly empty (重 虛)?"[5]

Ch'i Po answered: "When the constitution (the vigor of the pulse)
of the upper regions of the body is wanting and the 'cubit' pulse is
(also) wanting, it is called doubly empty."[6]

The Emperor asked: "How can this be cured?"

Ch'i Po answered: "The so-called wanting of vigor denotes an

4. Wang Ping explains: "Spring and Summer are influenced by Yang, the element of life;
therefore the mouth of the pulse is hot while there is cold within the 'cubit' pulse.   All
this causes compliance and order."

5. Wang Ping explains: "This question corresponds to the previous one: what is meant by
doubly full?"

6. Wang Ping explains: "This means that the 'cubit' pulse and the 'inch' pulse are both empty."

irregular condition. The emptiness of the 'cubit' pulse causes the movement of the pulse to be insufficient. The deficiency of the pulse does not come into appearance in the regions of Yin. And the procedure is as follows: When the pulse is smooth it means life, when the pulse is rough and uneven it means death."[7]

The Emperor asked: "When the breath is chilled and the upper regions of the body are scorched and when the pulse is full and solid, what does then happen?"[8]

Ch'i Po answered: "Fullness and smoothness mean life, but fullness and disorder mean death."

The Emperor asked: "When the pulse is full and complete and when hands and feet are chilly while the head is hot (feverish), what can be done?"

Ch'i Po answered: "Then it means that Spring and Fall bring life, while Winter and Summer bring death. When the pulse is excessive and harsh and uneven and when the entire body is hot (feverish) it means death."

The Emperor said: "When the phenomenon of the pulse is entirely complete[9] and the pulse is quick and of great firmness, but the 'cubit' pulse is rough and uneven[10] and not as it should be—and similar—, then order and compliance mean life while disorder and rebellion mean death."

And then the Emperor added: "How can one understand the saying: order means life (從 則 生) and disorder means death (逆 則 死)?"

Ch'i Po answered: "The so-called order means that hands and feet are warm. The so-called disorder means hands and feet are cold."

The Emperor asked: "When a child in arms has a disease with

7. Wang Ping explains: "When the 'inch' pulse is deficient, then the movements of the pulse become irregular; when the 'cubit' pulse is deficient, it causes the movement of the pulse to be insufficient."

8. Wang Ping supplies the emperor with a different question and Ch'i Po's answer seems to fit Wang Ping's question rather than the actual text: The Emperor asked: "It is said that when the vigor is heated and the pulse full this means 重 實 'doubly full.' When (the pulse is) smooth then there is compliance and order; when it is rough and uneven then there is disorder. Now, when the vigor is chilled and the pulse is full, can one call that too 'doubly full?' And what can one then do about the relation between smooth and rough, life and death, order and disorder?"

9. 其 形 盡 滿 .

10. Wang Ping quotes the 經 太 素 as saying 濇 作 滿 .

fever and the motions of the pulse are suspended and decreased what is the result?"

Ch'i Po answered: "If hands and feet are warm then it means life, when they are cold it means death."

The Emperor asked: "When a child in arms has a 'wind within' (中 風) and fever, when its breathing is troubled and it wheezes while resting its shoulders,[11] what is then the condition of the pulse?"

Ch'i Po answered: "When there is troubled breathing and wheezing while resting the shoulders, the pulse is large and full. When it is slow it means life; when it is rapid it means death."

The Emperor asked: "When while cleaning the bowels and while easing nature blood appears, what does this mean?"

Ch'i Po answered: "When the body is hot and feverish it means death; when the body is cool it means life."[12]

The Emperor asked: "When the cleaning of the bowels in descending carries white froth, what does this mean?"

Ch'i Po answered: "When the pulse is deep it means life; when it is superficial it means death."

The Emperor asked: "What does it mean when the cleaning of the bowels in descending carries bloody pus?"

Ch'i Po answered: "When the pulse is suspended and interrupted it means death; when it is smooth and large it means life."

The Emperor asked: "When in connection with the cleaning of the bowels the body is not hot (feverish) and the pulse is not suspended and interrupted, what will then occur?"

Ch'i Po answered: "When the pulse is smooth and large then it means life; when it is suspended and rough it means death. And one must also consider the season of each of the five viscera."[13]

The Emperor asked: "What can be done about madness and convulsions (癲 疾)?"

11. 喘 鳴 肩 息 .
12. Wang Ping explains: "Heat causes the spoilage of blood, therefore it means death. Coolness causes an advantageous atmosphere in regard to life, therefore it means life."
13. Wang Ping adds: "When the liver can be observed during the time of the celestial stems *kêng hsin* it means death; when the heart can be observed during the time of the celestial stems *jên kuei* it means death; when the lungs can be observed during the time of the celestial stems *ping ting* it means death; when the kidneys can be observed during the time of the celestial stems *wu chi* it means death; when the spleen can be observed during the time of the celestial stems *chia i* this means death. This means to take into consideration the seasons of the intestines."

Ch'i Po answered: "When the pulse strikes out in long beats and smoothly for a long time and then the beats of the pulse become smaller and hard on their own account, then a quick death will occur and no cure can be effected."

The Emperor asked: "What can be done when the pulse is insufficient or (too) full and when there are fits and madness?"

Ch'i Po replied: "When the pulse is wanting then the disease can be cured; when the pulse is (too) full then death will occur."

The Emperor asked: "If there is a digestive disease (of dissipation and exhaustion 消 癉), what can be done when the pulse is insufficient or when it is too full?"

Ch'i Po answered: "When the pulse is full and large, a chronic disease can be cured; when the pulse is suspended, small and hard then a chronic disease cannot be cured."

The Emperor said: "The laws of the body, the laws of the bones, the laws of the pulse and the laws of the extremities; how can these laws be known?"

Then the Emperor said: "During the height of Spring one should treat the veins and the arteries (經 絡), during the height of Summer one should treat the main arteries (經 俞), during the height of Fall one should treat the six bowels. In Winter, however, everything is closed and stopped up. And because everything is closed one should use medicine and only sparingly resort to acupuncture. (But) the so-called sparing use of acupuncture does not refer to the treatment of ulcers and deep seated abscesses,[14] for ulcers and abscesses must not be allowed to recur within a short time.

"When an ulcer develops without one's knowing its exact location (root) within the body, and when the physician then examines it with his hands, he is not able to achieve a result, for sometimes it is possible suddenly to feel the ulcer and sometimes the ulcer suddenly vanishes. When the physician applies acupuncture to a patient who suffers from ulcer, he pierces the hand three times in the region of the great Yin, (and that part of the 'sunlight' in the foot)[15] which

14. Wang Ping explains: "Although during the months of Winter the gates (of the body) are tightly closed, yet in regard to deep-seated ulcers and abscesses burning vapors within create a great moisture which cannot be quickly drained; and therefore the muscles become soft (suppurated) and the bones become putrid. Thus in spite of that which is fitting for the winter months, one must use acupuncture in order to open up and to get rid of the pus."

15. The part of the sentence in parentheses is taken from Wang Ping's commentary.

shows a bruise or a contusion (痏) and also the *ying mo* (纓 脉); and each of the parts he pierces twice.

"When the phenomenon of the ulcer causes the underarm (掖) to be very hot, the physician pierces three times [the region of] the lesser Yin of the foot.   And if then the heat does not cease he must pierce three times the region of the palm of the hand (?) (心 主); then he must also pierce three times the region of the great Yin of the hand, and the arteries and veins (*lo* vessels) between the shoulder and the back.

"When serious ulcers occur the muscles become soft and the pain is felt everywhere; perspiration comes out incessantly and the force of the bladder (胞 氣) becomes insufficient.   Then the physician must treat that part of the arteries that is hidden to the eyes.

"When the stomach of the patient feels full and cannot be pressed down with the hand, one should take the hand of the patient and treat it at [the region of] the great Yang, because the arteries and the veins of the great Yang are related to the inside of the stomach.

"When the ulcer occurs in that part of the lesser Yin which is three inches beside the backbone, the physician cures it by piercing this region five times with the round end (員) of the needle.

"When a patient suffers from a quick disorder (cholera) (霍 亂), the doctor cures it in the same part (as mentioned above), using the same instruments five times; and at the same time he also gives treatment by piercing three times in [the region of] the 'sunlight' within the foot and in the upper part of the region of the lesser Yin.

"When a patient suffers from fits and sudden alarms (癇 驚), the physician treats his pulse five times,[16] and at the same time the physician must pierce five times each hand of the patient in the [region of the] great Yin; and he must also pierce five times the arteries of the hands in the [region of the] great Yin as well as in the [region of the] lesser Yin; he must pierce once the arteries and veins and also once the [region of the] 'sunlight' in the foot, and finally he must pierce three times the part which is five inches above the ankle.

"Generally one can cure digestive diseases, strokes, and falling prostrate, paralysis on one side, impotence, and that fullness of vigor which gives rise to disorders.   When these diseases occur with

16. Wang Ping explains: "This means the pulse of the *Yang ling ch'üan* (陽 陵 泉), which is located within the upper outer concave below the knee."

wealthy people, then they are ailments caused by rich fare (高=膏粱). When there are divisions, blockages, closings, and cuttings off, and movement ceases above and below, then there are diseases brought about by violent (sudden) stress.

"One-sided deafness, blockages and closures, and lack of movement cause the inner vigor to become heated and weak. Disorders of the interior, the exterior, and the middle are diseases caused by the wind. Therefore they are manifested by a protracted state of emaciation. Lameness and cold soles of the feet are diseases which are caused by wind and dampness (風 濕)."

The Emperor said: "When the yellow ulcer becomes violently painful, the patient will have fits and be delirious and finally act contrary to what is natural.[17] Then the five viscera are not healthy; the six hollow organs are closed and barred to that which is produced; the head aches; the ear hears sounds; the nine orifices do not function beneficially with that which is produced by the stomach and the intestines."

17. 黃疸暴 痛 癲疾 厥 狂 久 逆 之 所生 也.

29. *Treatise on the Region of the Great Yin and on the Region of the 'Sunlight'*

The Yellow Emperor asked: "The great Yin and the 'sunlight' are related to the reaction of pulse of the spleen and the pulse of the stomach. When a disease arises and this system is changed, what then?"

Ch'i Po answered: "Yin and Yang have a different position; it changes in regard to deficiency and fullness; it changes in regard to disorder and compliance.[1] Whether they correspond to the inside, or whether they correspond to the outside, this relation is not the same; therefore the diseases (from any of these sources) have different designations (名)."[2]

1 Wang Ping explains: "Both spleen and stomach, viscera and bowels, belong respectively to the element of the earth; when one falls ill this system will be changed, therefore the physician inquires into the dissimilitude."

2. Wang Ping explains: "The spleen, one of the viscera, belongs to Yin; the stomach, one of the bowels, belongs to Yang; the pulse of Yang lead downwards; the pulse of Yin leads upwards; the pulse of Yang corresponds to the outside; the pulse of Yin corresponds to the inside. Therefore it is said: the (Yin and Yang) do not correspond to the same (factors) and their diseases have different names."

The Emperor said: "I should like to be informed about the difference of the symptoms (forms)."

Ch'i Po answered: "Yang is related to the heavenly atmosphere and it controls the outside. Yin is related to the climate of the earth and it controls the inside. Thus the way of Yang is fullness and the way of Yin is emptiness.[3] To rebel and to transgress against the wind will bring about weakness and suffering from bad influences. This will cause suffering to the element of Yang (陽 受 之). Eating and drinking without moderation, irregular hours in rising and resting will cause suffering to the element of Yin (陰 受 之).[4] When the element of Yang suffers then the six bowels are affected. When the element of Yin suffers then the five viscera are affected.

"When the six hollow organs are affected, then the heat of the body is unseasonable (irregular), and even lying down causes pain at the time of exhalation in the upper part of the body. When the five viscera are filled up (膩=閩) and stuffed, the descent is blocked and closed, which causes the food to leak out in the lower part of the body. This, if protracted, causes the bowels to be washed out.[5]

"The throat is related to the heavenly atmosphere and the blockages are related to the climate of the earth; thus Yang suffers through the wind, while Yin suffers through damp air.

"The influence of Yin begins at the foot and in ascending reaches the head, while in descending it follows the arm up to the beginning of the fingers. The influence of Yang begins at the hand and in ascending reaches the head, while in descending it goes down to the foot.

"Thus a disease of the element of Yang ascends until it reaches the utmost height and then it descends; while a disease of the element of Yin descends to the lowest point and then ascends. Hence an injury suffered through the wind will first ascend when contracted. An injury suffered through humidity will first descend when contracted."

The Emperor said: "When the spleen is sick, the four extremities cannot be used. How is that?"

Ch'i Po answered: "The four extremities are closely related to the

3. Wang Ping explains: "These are the so-called changes in regard to deficiency and fullness."
4. Wang Ping explains: "This is the so-called relationship between Yin and Yang: whether they correspond to the inside or whether they correspond to the outside."
5. Wang Ping explains: "This is the so-called difference of the relations and explains the different designations of the diseases."

stomach, but they cannot communicate with the stomach directly.[6] The spleen is an essential factor and it creates the connection.[7] Now, when the spleen is sick it cannot cause the stomach to create secretions; the four limbs do not receive nourishment (稟) through the vigor of water and grain. Vigor deteriorates daily; the way of the pulse is not advantageous; the muscles, the bones and the flesh, they all do not have the vigor which is necessary to life, therefore they cannot be used."

The Emperor asked: "Why is it that the spleen does not control (is not related to 主) one season?"[8]

Ch'i Po answered: "The spleen corresponds to the earth. It regulates the center, that which is constant. This serves to extend the four seasons. Each of the four viscera is entrusted with eighteen days of regulation, but they must not alone control the seasons. The spleen, one of the viscera, manifests itself constantly in the essence (secretions) of the stomach and the soil.

"Everything in creation is produced by the soil, and is then governed by Heaven and Earth. Thus above and below, the head and the foot, cannot be directly influenced by the (temperature of) the four seasons."

The Emperor said: "The spleen and the stomach have a thin membrane (膜) that joins them together. Which then has the power to cause the procedure of the fluid secretions?"

Ch'i Po answered: "The Great Yin of the foot means (relates to) the three Yin. Its communication by way of the stomach is subject to the spleen and is connected with the throat; thus it is the great Yin which causes the communication to the three parts of Yin. The region of the 'sunlight' in the stomach is the outer part of the spleen.[9]

"The five viscera and the six hollow organs are like an ocean (a reservoir 海). They also serve to transport vigor to the three

6. Wang Ping quotes 按 太 素 to say 至 經 to mean 徑 至.

7. Wang Ping explains: "The vigor of the spleen distributes and transforms the water and the grain into essences and secretions which reach the four limbs and give them nourishment."

8. Wang Ping explains: "The liver is related to Spring; the heart is related to Summer; the lungs are related to Fall; the kidneys are related to Winter. Each of the four viscera has one exact season to which it corresponds, but the spleen does not have an exact season to which it is related."

9. Wang Ping explains: "The spleen belongs to Yin and the stomach belongs to Yang. The spleen belongs to the inside, the stomach belongs to the outside; their respective position is different, but they assist each other."

regions of Yang. The viscera and the hollow organs, in reliance upon their direct communication, receive vigor from the region of the 'sunlight'. Thus they cause the stomach to transport its fluid secretions.

"When the four limbs do not receive vigor and nourishment (water and grain), there will be daily increasing deterioration.[10] The principle of Yin does not work beneficially; the muscles, the bones, and the flesh do not have the vigor which is needed for life, and hence the (four limbs) cannot be used."

10. Wang Ping explains: "Here is again repeated the illustration that the spleen is directly responsible for the proper condition of the four limbs."

30. *Treatise on the Distribution of the Pulse of the 'Sunlight'*

The Yellow Emperor asked: "If the pulse of the 'sunlight' within the foot is sick, man is hurt by fire, and when he hears the tone of wood he is startled. But although this startles him, bells and drums do not cause excitement to him. But how is it that when the patient hears the sound of wood he is startled?"

Ch'i Po answered: "The pulse of the 'sunlight' is the pulse of the stomach. (The element of) the stomach is the earth. Thus when one hears the tone of wood and is startled, the earth has injured the wood."[1]

The emperor said: "Excellent; but what about the injurious fire?"

Ch'i Po answered: "[*Yang Ming*] the region of the 'sunlight' is in close relation with the pulse of the flesh. If within the vigor of the blood there resides evil there is heat. When the heat is great then there is hurtful fire."

The Emperor asked: "How does it hurt man?"

Ch'i Po answered: "If [the region of] the 'sunlight' is deficient then panting will occur and distress. When there is distress it is hurtful to man."

The Emperor said: "I wonder whether breathlessness results in death or whether it results in life."

Ch'i Po answered: "When there are deficiencies and blockages in the circulation between the viscera, then death follows. When the circulation is not impeded, life follows."

1. Wang Ping explains that the Book of Yin and Yang says: "the tree (wood) is destroyed by the soil, thus the soil injures the tree (wood)."

The Emperor said: "Excellent! When the illness is grave, should then the clothes be cast aside and should one walk about, and should one ascend the heights chanting songs or is it best to fast for one day? And all those who transgress a wall or who dwell upon heights, are they not able to maintain their original constitution, and can the disease come back to them?"

Ch'i Po answered: "The four limbs all originate from the element of Yang. When Yang is flourishing then the four limbs are in a state of sufficiency, and when there exists this state of sufficiency one can ascend the heights."

The Emperor asked: "Should the clothes be cast aside?"

Ch'i Po answered: "When the heat is sufficient for the body, the clothes can be cast aside if one intends to walk."

The Emperor asked: "Those (people) who tell lies, and scold and curse and do not shirk treating their relatives distantly, and yet chant songs—what [can you tell] about them?"

Ch'i Po answered: "When the element of Yang is plentiful, it causes man to tell lies; he does not shirk treating his relatives distantly, and he does not have a desire for food. Since he does not have a desire for food his actions become reckless and disorderly."

Book 9

31. *Treatise on the Hot Sickness*

THE Yellow Emperor asked: "Now what is the hot sickness (熱 病)? It belongs to the class of 'the injuries of the cold' (typhoid fevers 傷 寒). They are either cured or followed by death. Their death always takes the period of six or seven days, their improvement takes ten days. Can it also take more? I do not know the explanation and desire to know the foundation."

Ch'i Po answered: "The great Yang[1] is everything that is connected with Yang. Its pulse is connected with the store-house of the wind[2] and therefore it causes the entire Yang to be related to the force of life.

"When man is injured by the cold [suffers from a gastric (?) fever], then a disease with heat (fever) is caused. But although the fever is great death does not occur. When both (the viscera and the bowels)[3] are affected by the cold (fever) and become ill, death cannot be avoided."

The Emperor said: "I should like to be informed of their appearance."[4]

Ch'i Po answered: "On the first day the 'injury of the cold' is received by [the region of] the great Yang.[5] Therefore head and neck are in pain; the waist and the back become rigid. On the second day [the region of] the 'sunlight' receives it [the disease]. The 'sunlight' controls the flesh, its pulse supports the nose, and is connected with the eyes. Thus the body is hot (feverish), the eyes ache, the nose is dry [and parched], and the patient finds it impossible to rest. On the third day [the region of] the lesser Yang

1. Wang Ping explains that 巨 陽 is equal to 太 陽.
2. Wang Ping explains that the store-house of the wind (風 府) is a sinus in the body, located in the nape of the neck.
3. The words in parentheses are added by Wang Ping.
4. Wang Ping explains this to mean: "What is the appearance when not both, the viscera and the bowels, are affected?"
5. Wang Ping explains: "The pulse of the great Yang is located within the skin and the body hair; therefore the 'injury of the cold' is on the first day received by the region of the great Yang."

receives it. The [region of the] lesser Yang controls the gall bladder. Its pulse follows the flanks and is connected with the ears. Thus the ribs and the chest are painful and the ear becomes deaf. Now the three [regions of] Yang, the arteries and the veins, they all have received the disease, but it has not yet entered into the viscera;[6] therefore one can produce perspiration and terminate it. On the fourth day [the region of] the great Yang receives the disease. The [region of the] great Yang leads into the interior of the stomach and is connected with the throat, thus the stomach becomes replete (full) and the throat becomes dry [and parched]. On the fifth day [the region of] the lesser Yin receives the disease. The pulse of [the region of] the lesser Yin penetrates to the kidneys and is connected with the lungs, and it is also connected with the root of the tongue. Thus the mouth is dry and the tongue is parched and thirsty. On the sixth day the [region of the] absolute Yin receives the disease. The pulse of [the region of] the absolute Yin passes through to the sex organs and is connected with the liver; the result is an affliction of fullness, the scrotum shrinks. Now the three regions of Yin and the three regions of Yang, the five viscera and the six bowels have all received the disease; and the blood and the vital substances no longer circulate in the five viscera. Then death follows.

"When not both [the viscera and the bowels][7] are affected by the cold, the sickness of the great Yang improves somewhat[8] on the seventh day and the head aches less. On the eighth day the 'sunlight' improves, and the body becomes less hot [feverish]. On the ninth day the lesser Yang becomes less sick, the ears become less deaf and the patient can hear a little. On the tenth day the great Yin becomes less sick, the [swelling of the] stomach is reduced, and the patient thinks of food and drink as he was formerly used to do.[9] On the eleventh day the region of the lesser Yin becomes less sick, thirst and dryness of the tongue cease [to bother him], and sneezing

6. Wang Ping explains: "Because the evil is on the outside one can bring about perspiration." Wang Ping quotes several references according to which it should read 'bowels' (腑) instead of viscera (臟).

7. 兩 感 liang-kan may also mean a particularly severe form of the "cold fever." See Franz Hübotter: Die Medizin zu Beginn des XX Jahrhunderts und ihr historischer Entwicklungsgang. Leipzig, 1929. (Chinabibliothek der "Asia Major" Bd. 1), p. 93.

8. Wang Ping adds: "The utmost point of Yang is reached and Yin receives the disease."

9. 如 故 則 思 飲 食 .

ensues. On the twelfth day the absolute Yin becomes less sick, the scrotum slackens, the [swelling of the] stomach is reduced, and all the great (evil)[10] vapors depart; and after one day the sickness is improved."

The Emperor said: "What can be done in regard to treatment?"

Ch'i Po answered: "The method of curing the 'injury of the cold' is to establish communication between the system of the viscera and the vascular system, and then the illness will weaken day by day. When the patient has been ill for less than three days, one can bring about perspiration [and thus terminate the disease], and that is all. When a patient has been ill for more than three days, one can bring about (abdominal) dispersion!"

The Emperor asked: "When the hot sickness comes to an end and is cured, why does there sometimes remain [some elements of illness]?"

Ch'i Po answered: "All these remnants of illness are caused when the patient was made to eat too much while the fever was high; then there are remnants. All of this means that the illness has retreated but the heat (fever) is still within the body, because the energies of the foods attack each other and two elements of heat join together so that the fever (heat) remains."

The Emperor said: "Well, but how can you cure the illness of the remnants?"

Ch'i Po answered: "It is by determining its fullness and deficiency and by harmonizing its opposition and attraction that we can cause it to be cured."

The Emperor said: "How can you apprehend and prevent the sickness of heat (熱 病)?"

Ch'i Po answered: "When the illness of heat shows little improvement and when (the patient) eats meat, then there will be a relapse; when the patient eats too much there will be a remnant. This [knowledge] is its prevention."

The Emperor said: "When the illness is caused by the cold, both [inside and outside] the region of the great Yang and the region of the lesser Yin are affected on the first day of the illness; then there will be a headache, the mouth is parched and very uncomfortable.[11]

10. The word in parentheses was added from the commentary. Wang Ping explains: "Because the evil vapors depart improvement can take place."
11. Wang Ping says: 煩 滿 should mean 渴, thirsty.

On the second day of the illness the region of the 'sunlight' and the great Yin are all affected; then the stomach feels full, the body feels hot, and the patient does not want food and he speaks deliriously. On the third day of the illness the region of the lesser Yang and of the absolute Yin are affected, then the ear is deaf and the scrotum shrinks and becomes deficient (厥=闕); water and broth cannot enter, the patient cannot recognize other people and on the sixth day he will die."[12]

The Emperor said: "When the five viscera are injured and there is no flow within the six bowels, and when the blood and the vital substances do not proceed, how can the patient be like this for three days and die only then? (Why will he die only after three days?)"

Ch'i Po answered: "The 'sunlight' is the superior of the twelve main vessels. The patient's vigor of blood is still strong so that he can [live, but] not recognize anyone, but three days later this vigor will be exhausted and then he dies.

"In general those patients who suffer from an 'injury of the cold' are revived. Those who [fall ill] before summer solstice have the warm sickness; those who fall ill after summer solstice have the (very) hot sickness. This heat should be treated with perspiration, so that everything is emitted without clogging."[13]

12. Wang Ping explains: "The great Yang and the lesser Yin serve as coat and lining (outside and inside); the 'sunlight' and the great Yin serve as coat and lining; the lesser Yang and the absolute Yin serve as coat and lining; therefore when (outside and inside) are both affected by cold atmosphere, they suffer (receive the evil) together."

13. Wang Ping explains: "Those who are injured slightly by the cold in winter will develop a warm sickness (溫 病) before summer solstice. Those who are injured severely by the cold in winter will develop a hot (暑 病) sickness after summer."

32. *Treatise on the Method of Applying Acupuncture to the Illness of the Heat*

When the illness of the heat (hot disease) (熱 病) is located in the liver, at first the urine becomes yellow, then the stomach hurts, the patient wishes to lie down, and his body is hot (feverish). The elements of heat conflict within the body and cause delirious speech and sudden starts during the sleep; the ribs and flanks are full of pain, hands and feet are restless, and the patient cannot lie down peacefully.

When the region of the celestial stems *kêng hsin* is heavy, the region of the celestial stems *chia i* produces great perspiration; when the breath is in disorder the region of the celestial stems *kêng hsin* brings death.[1]

One should apply acupuncture to the foot at the region of the absolute Yin and the lesser Yang.[2]   When one acts against this then there follows dizziness, and the pulse moves heavily within the head.

When the illness of the heat is located in the heart, there is no joy; after several days there is fever.[3]   When the elements of heat conflict [within the body], they cause sudden pains at the heart, hidden troubles, dangerous vomiting, headaches, red complexion, and lack of perspiration.

When the region of the celestial stems *jên kuei* is heavy, the region of *ping ting* produces much perspiration.   When the breath is in disorder then the region of *jên kuei* brings death.[4]   (Then) one should apply acupuncture to the foot at the region of the lesser Yin and the great Yang.[5]

When the spleen has the illness of the heat, then, at first, the head becomes heavy, the cheeks are in pain and [the heart] is afflicted. The complexion (color) turns green; there is a desire to vomit and the body is hot.   When the elements of heat conflict [within the body], then the loins hurt and cannot be used for the purpose of looking down or up, the stomach is full and there is a leakage and both the jaws hurt.

When the region of the celestial stems *chia i* is heavy, the region of *wu chi* produces much perspiration.   When the breath is in disorder, then the region of *chia i* brings death.[6]   (Then) one should

1. Wang Ping explains: "The liver rules over wood, the celestial stems *kêng hsin* correspond to metal; metal destroys wood, thus it is heavy and death comes from the celestial stems *kêng hsin*.   *Chia i* corresponds to wood, thus much perspiration comes forth from *chia i*."
2. Wang Ping explains: "The absolute Yin is connected with the pulse of the liver; the lesser Yang is connected with the pulse of the gall bladder."
3. Wang Ping explains: "The atmosphere of the disease of the heart enters into the arteries and veins, then the spirit is not peaceful and orderly."
4. Wang Ping explains: "The heart rules over fire; the celestial stems *jên kuei* correspond to water; water extinguishes fire, thus it is heavy and death comes from *jên kuei*; *ping ting* corresponds to wood, thus much perspiration comes from *ping ting*."
5. The lesser Yin is connected with the pulse of the heart; the great Yang is connected with the pulse of the small intestines.
6. The spleen rules over the earth; the celestial stems *chia i* are connected with wood.   Wood

apply acupuncture to the foot at the regions of the great Yin and the 'sunlight.'

When the lungs suffer from the illness of the heat, then at first, when [the body is] brought in contact with cold, there is a startling sensation, goose pimples spring up and an aversion (arises) towards cold wind and cold air; the upper side of the tongue turns yellow and the body becomes hot. When the elements of heat conflict within the body, there is heavy breathing and panting and the pain is felt throughout the thorax and the breast; the back of the patient cannot rest comfortably, he has headaches and is unable to endure his suffering (physically unfit); perspiration appears and he has chills.

When the region of the celestial stems *ping ting* is heavy, the region of *kêng hsin* produces much perspiration. When the breath is in disorder the region of *ping ting* brings death.' (Then) one should apply acupuncture to the hands at the region of the great Yin and the 'sunlight', and the blood will gush forth as though a large vessel had been placed there.

When the kidneys suffer from the illness of heat, then at first, the waist (loins 腰) is in pain, the thighbone (coccyx 骱) has muscular pains; there is suffering of thirst [in spite of] frequent drinking, and the body is hot.[8] When then the elements of the heat conflict with each other, then the neck hurts and becomes rigid, the part of the coccyx feels cold and painful, the part below the foot (the sole) feels hot, and the patient cannot speak. If the reverse [of the condition previously described] is the case, it is the neck that feels pain and is stiff and uncomfortable.

When the region of the celestial stems *wu chi* feels heavy, the region of *jên kuei* produces much perspiration. When the breath is in disorder then the region of *wu chi* brings death. (Then) one

---

cuts into the earth, therefore wood is mighty and death comes from *chia i*. *Wu chi* corresponds to earth, therefore much perspiration comes from *wu chi*.

7. The lungs correspond to metal; the celestial stems *ping ting* are connected with fire; fire melts metal, therefore fire is mighty and death comes from the region of *ping ting*. The celestial stems *kêng hsin* correspond to metal, therefore great perspiration comes from *kêng hsin*.

8. The kidneys correspond to water; the celestial stems *wu chi* are connected with the earth; the earth punishes (absorbs) the water, therefore it is mighty, and death comes from the region of *wu chi*. The celestial stems *jên kuei* correspond to water, therefore much perspiration comes from *jên kuei*.

should apply acupuncture to the feet at the regions of the lesser Yin and the great Yang.[9]

All [the hot diseases] which must be cured by perspiration should be cured on a special day by much perspiration.

The symptoms of the sickness of the heat, located in the liver, are that the left side of the jaw first turns red. The symptoms of the sickness of the heat, located in the heart, are that the complexion first turns red. The symptoms of the sickness of the heat, located in the spleen, are that the nose first turns red. The symptoms of the sickness of the heat, located in the lungs, are that the right side of the jaw first turns red. The symptoms of the sickness of the heat, located in the kidneys, are that the chin first turns red. Thus, although the disease has not yet developed, one can observe it by the redness of the complexion and one can apply acupuncture. This means: 'to treat the disease when it has not yet developed.' When one of the diseases caused by heat arises, it takes one period (期)[10] to be terminated.

The heat disease begins [at a certain part of the body] and is symbolized (by two of the ten celestial stems), and it will be cured at the date (which coincides with the two celestial stems). If this disease is treated at the opposite[11] region [from where it arose], it takes three cycles of the celestial stems to cure it. If it is again treated in the opposite way death will result. All [the heat diseases] that must be cured by perspiration should be cured on a special day by much perspiration.

In order to cure every heat disease, one should first prescribe potions of cold water and then acupuncture. The patient should wear thin clothing and should be stretched out in a cool place, and when his body becomes cold one should cease with the application of acupuncture.[12]

9. The region of the lesser Yin is connected with the pulse of the kidneys; the region of the great Yang is connected with the pulse of the bladder.

10. 期 means a day of great perspiration. (Explained by Wang Ping.)

11. Wang Ping explains: 反, opposite, means to take the opposite of the atmosphere, as though a disease of the liver were to be treated at the spleen, and a disease of the lungs were treated at the liver. All this would be the opposite treatment of the atmosphere of the five viscera.

12. When the cold water is in the stomach, the atmosphere of Yang is abundant on the outside. Therefore one gives potions of cold water and then applies acupuncture; then the heat will withdraw and coolness will develop, and when the body is cool one should cease to puncture.

At the occasion of a disease of the heat at first the thorax and the flanks are in pain, and the hands and the feet become restless. Then one should apply acupuncture to the foot at [the region of] the lesser Yang and supplement the foot at [the region of] the great Yin. When the disease is severe one should apply fifty-nine needles (punctuations).

When the disease of the heat begins with pains at the hands and the arms, one should apply acupuncture to the hands at [the region of] the 'sunlight' and the great Yin, and cease when the patient begins to perspire.

When the disease of the heat begins at the head, one should apply acupuncture to the neck at [the region of] the great Yang and cease when the patient begins to perspire.

When the disease of the heat begins at the vessels of the foot (足 經), then one should apply acupuncture to the foot at [the region of] the 'sunlight' and cease when the patient begins to perspire.

When the disease of the heat first strikes at the important parts of the body, the bones ache and the ears turn deaf; then one should apply acupuncture to [the region of] the lesser Yin. When the disease is grave one should make fifty-nine punctures.

When the disease of the heat first causes dizziness and confused vision and fever, and then the flanks and the thorax become full, one should apply acupuncture to the foot at [the regions of] the lesser Yin and the lesser Yang and to the pulse of the great Yang.

When the color (appearance, complexion) is [bright] and flourishing, then upon examination [one finds] that the bones suffer from the disease of the heat; the flourishing physical appearance is not evenly blended, and it is said that (although) presently there should be perspiration one must wait for the proper time.[13]

When conflict in regard to the pulse of the absolute Yin becomes visible, the date of death will not exceed three days. When the disease of the heat is within the body, it comes in contact with the kidneys (finding expression in the pulse and the appearance of the lesser Yang).[14] If then the pulse and the appearance show flourish-

13. Wang Ping explains: "This means: in the case of a disease of the liver one must wait for the celestial stems *chia i*; in the case of a disease of the heart one must wait for the celestial stems *ping ting*;" etc.

14. The New Commentary continues: "When the kidneys are hot they are injured and therefore death occurs." The following six characters, 少 陽 之 脉 色 也 , were added by Wang Ping and are considered unnecessary by later commentators.

ing cheeks, it is manifest that the disease of the heat is located in the muscles; the flourishing (physical appearance) is not evenly blended, and it is said that, although there should be perspiration presently, one should wait for the proper time.

When conflict in regard to the pulse of the lesser Yin becomes visible, then the date of death will not exceed three days. The point of acupuncture which lies in the part beneath the three vertebral sections of the backbone is related to the heat in the stomach, which is one of the heat diseases. If the heat is within the diaphragm the point of acupuncture lies beneath the fourth section of the backbone. If the heat is within the liver the point of acupuncture lies beneath the fifth section of the backbone. If the heat is within the spleen the point of acupuncture lies beneath the sixth section of the backbone. If the heat is within the kidneys the point of acupuncture lies beneath the seventh section of the backbone, which (also) influences the coccyx. The space between the three sections of the backbone above the neck should (also) be used for acupuncture.[15]

If the heat resides beneath the cheeks at the cheekbones it causes a severe disease of the bowels (大 瘕). If the lower teeth shake it means that the abdomen is full. If the disease lies behind the cheekbones it causes pains in the ribs, because the part above the cheeks is related to the diaphragm.

15. 項 上 三 椎 陷 者 中 也 .

熱 病, the "heat disease," "hot disease" or "disease of the heat," is one of the five types of feverish diseases which are enumerated in the *Nan Ching*, chapter 58. The other four are: 中 風, "the internal wind," 傷 寒, "the cold disease" or "the disease of the cold," 濕 溫, "the humid lukewarm [disease]," and 溫 病, "the lukewarm disease."

33. *Commentary on the Treatise on the 'Warm Illness'*

The Yellow Emperor asked: "There are 'warm illnesses' (病 溫); although patients perspire the fever (heat) returns abruptly, and although the pulse is hasty and rapid it does not cause perspiration. The patients become weakened and mad, and it is said that they are not able to eat. What is the meaning (name) of this disease?"

Ch'i Po answered: "The meaning of this disease is that Yin and Yang are interlocked, and when they are interlocked it means death."

Huang Ti said: "I desire to hear it explained."

Ch'i Po answered: "The life of all those people who perspire springs from grain, and grain is produced from (pure) essence. Now, when the evil influences are interlocked in battle with the bones and the flesh, then perspiration should come forth so that the evil (airs) remove themselves and the pure essence excels. When the pure essence excels then the patient should be able to eat and the heat will not return. When the heat returns it means that there is (still) evil air, but when there is perspiration it means purity. Now, when perspiration appears and the heat returns at once, it means that the evil is victorious. Then the patient is not able to eat and the essence is not helpful (in producing perspiration).

"When an illness[1] persists, man's allotted span of life will forthwith be exhausted and he may collapse. Furthermore in the 'treatise on the heat'[2] it is said: 'When perspiration appears and the pulse is yet hasty and full, death will follow.' Now, the pulse does not respond to the perspiration and the disease cannot be overcome; thus death can be understood.

"Those who speak nonsense (are delirious) have lost their determination, and those who have lost their determination will die. Now, we have seen three (kinds of) death, but we have not seen one (kind of) life.[3] It is difficult to cure one who is bound to die."

Huang Ti said: "The body is afflicted by diseases where perspiration appears and where (the patient) is troubled by fullness. This trouble of fullness does not cause the perspiration to be released; how does it affect the illness?"

Ch'i Po answered: "When perspiration appears and the body is hot there will be insanity (paralysis 瘋). When perspiration appears and the trouble of fullness is not dispersed, there will be convulsions (痸). The names of the disease indicate paralysis and convulsions."

Huang Ti said: "I desire to know it completely."

Ch'i Po answered: "The great Yang controls the breath, therefore it is the first to be subjected to evil influences. The lesser Yin and the great Yang constitute the outside and the inside. In order to get hold of the heat one must follow it upwards, and when one follows upwards then one (reaches) the convulsions."

1. 甲乙經 says: "When the heat persists."
2. The treatise on the heat means: 上古熱論 .
3. Wang Ping says: "When perspiration comes forth and the pulse is violent and full, this is one kind of death. When one cannot overcome the disease, it is the second kind of death. When one is delirious and loses one's determination, it is the third kind of death."

The Yellow Emperor said: "What remedy can there (be applied) for the treatment?"

Ch'i Po answered: "One must apply acupuncture to the inside and the outside, and as drink one must give a dose of hot liquid as medicine."[4]

The Yellow Emperor asked: "Does not the troublesome wind[5] cause illness?"

Ch'i Po answered: "The troublesome wind affects, as a rule, the place beneath the lungs, bringing about illness in this place, and causing man to be well able to look upwards but to be confused when he looks downwards. Saliva and mucus appear; evil winds then bring about chills, and this causes the illness of the troublesome wind."

The Yellow Emperor asked: "Is there any way to cure this?"

Ch'i Po answered: "In order to help (restore) elasticity the region of the great Yang must conduct the secretions (essence), and if within three to five days there are no secretions, then, after seven days, a cough will come with green and yellow mucus, in appearance like pus and in size like a small ball; it will come from within the mouth and from within the nose; and if it does not come out, it will injure the lungs, and if it injures the lungs, death will result."

The Emperor said: "There is a disease which paralyses the kidneys, the surface and the bowels are sick and burning, and there is an injurious obstacle in regard to speech. Can one in such a case apply acupuncture or not?"

Ch'i Po answered: "When there is deficiency one should not apply acupuncture. When one should not apply acupuncture and does yet apply it, the breath will be (exhausted) at the extreme point."

The Emperor asked: "What is it about this extreme point?"

Ch'i Po answered: "At this extreme point there is of necessity shortness of breath and periods of fever. These periods of fever come from the thorax and ascend the back to its highest point, the head. Sweat appears, the hands are hot, the mouth is dry as though it were thirsty, the urine is yellow; there are swellings underneath the eyes; there are sounds within the stomach, the body (is heavy

4. Wang Ping says: "One drains (the region of) the great Yang and one supplements (the region of) the lesser Yin. To give hot liquids to drink means to stop the disorder from reaching the kidneys."

5. 勞 風.

and) suffers when walking, the menses do not come, there is trouble and lack of ability to eat, and inability to stand up straight and to lie down. When one stands up straight or lies down there is coughing. The name of this disease is "wind and water" and it is discussed in the treatise of the 'methods of acupuncture.' "[6]

The Emperor said: "I wish to hear you describe it."

Ch'i Po answered: "At the point where the evil flows together, there is, of necessity, emptiness (want) of breath. When Yin is empty, Yang must of necessity unite. Therefore there arises shortness of breath and periods of fever, and perspiration appears. The urine is yellow and there is little of it, and there is heat within the stomach. The patient cannot stand up straight and within the stomach there is no harmony (order). When the patient stands up or lies down, there is a severe cough which ascends and oppresses the lungs. All this is water and breath, and minute swellings can first be observed underneath the eyes."

The Emperor said: "What is the explanation for this?"

Ch'i Po answered: "Water is Yin and (the region) underneath the eyes is also Yin, and the highest (extreme) point of the stomach is the place where Yin resides. Hence water is within the stomach and must, of necessity, cause the swellings beneath the eyes. The true (real) breath ascends in opposition, hence the mouth and the tongue are dry, the patient cannot rest, neither can he stand up nor lie down. If he stands up or lies down he coughs and pure water appears. All this water means sickness; hence he cannot rest. If he sleeps he is (easily) startled, and if he is startled he coughs heavily. There are sounds within the stomach and the disease originates within the stomach. The weakened spleen causes trouble, the patient cannot eat and the food cannot descend; the ducts leading to the stomach are severed. The body is heavy and suffers when walking about, (for) the pulse of the stomach is in the foot. The menses do not come and the pulse of the thorax is obstructed. The pulse of the thorax belongs to the heart and the blood vessels lie within the thorax. If now the breath rises it oppresses the lungs and the heart, but then the breath cannot descend and circulate, hence the menses cannot come."

The Emperor said: "Excellent!"

6. Wang Ping says that the volume by the name of "Method of Acupuncture" is now a lost classic.

34. *Treatise on Rebellion and Harmony*

The Yellow Emperor asked: "Man's body is never constantly warm, nor is it constantly hot. Is it because of the heat that afflictions of deficiencies arise?"

Ch'i Po answered: "When Yin is wanting, Yang excels, hence it is then the heat that causes afflictions and deficiencies."

The Yellow Emperor asked: "When man's body is unclothed there are chills, (although) within (the body) there is no cold air. Are chills produced from within?"

Ch'i Po answered: "In cases where man is prone to numbness in breathing (痺 氣), there is shortness of Yang and an abundance of Yin. Hence the body is cold as though it had come out of the water."

The Yellow Emperor said: "Man has four extremities. When they are hot and meet with a wind, do they not become chilled as though they had been cauterized or burnt?"

Ch'i Po said: "Such persons have a deficiency of Yin and an abundance of Yang. The two Yang combine and Yin is insufficient. An insufficient quantity of water cannot exterminate a great fire and thus Yang governs alone. (Yet) if it governs alone it cannot continue to grow. If it excels in solitude it will cease (to exist). If it meets with a wind and is affected as though it were cauterized or burnt, then man's flesh must melt (disintegrate)."

The Yellow Emperor asked: "In such cases where man has a cold body (chills), if one heats it with fire one cannot make it hot; if one clothes it heavily one cannot make it warm; what can one do to keep it from freezing?"

Ch'i Po answered: "Man's original constitution overcomes the force of the kidneys by the application of water. When the great Yang deteriorates, the fat of the kidneys dries up and does not develop. (But) one (part of) water does not overcome two (parts of) fire; the kidneys are water.[1] Although there is life within the bones, the kidneys cannot live; hence the marrow cannot be complete and thus the chills reach the bones, but cannot freeze them.

"The liver is one (part of) Yang; the heart is two (parts of) Yang. The kidneys are isolated among the viscera. One (part of) water cannot overcome two (parts of) fire, hence it cannot congeal. The

---

1. The kidneys belong to the element of water.

name of the disease is 'numbness of the bones'(骨 痺).   This happens when people have crooked joints."[2]

The Yellow Emperor said: "If man has afflictions of the bones, although fleecy clothes are close (to his body) and yet he has afflictions, how does one call this illness?"[3]

Ch'i Po answered: "When there is blood there is deficiency, when there are vital essences then there is fullness.   When there is a deficiency because of the blood then there is numbness.   When there is fullness because of the vital essences, the (limbs; the body?) cannot be used.   When the blood and the vital essences are both deficient, then everything is without sensation and, as before, the flesh loses its function.   Man's body does not have any coordination and death follows within a day."

The Yellow Emperor said: "Man is afflicted when he cannot rest and when his breathing has a sound (is noisy)—or when he cannot rest and his breathing is without any sound.   He may rise and rest (his habits of life may be) as of old and his breathing is noisy; he may have his rest and his exercise and his breathing is troubled (wheezing, panting); or he may not get any rest and be unable to walk about and his breathing is troubled.   There are those who do not get a rest and those who rest and yet have troubled breathing. Is all this caused by the viscera?   I desire to hear about their causes."

Ch'i Po answered: "Those who do not rest and whose breathing is noisy have disorders in the region of Yang Ming (the 'sunlight'). The Yang of the foot in descending causes the present disturbance and in ascending it causes the breathing to be noisy.   The pulse of the stomach is located in the region of the 'sunlight'.   The stomach is the ocean of the five viscera.[4]   If the breath (of the stomach) does not function there is a disorder in [the region of] the 'sunlight' and it cannot follow its course; the consequence is inability to rest.   In ancient classics it is said: 'If there is no harmony within the stomach, there is no peace (contentment, comfort, ease).'

"Hence if the habits of life are as usual and the breathing is noisy, then the veins of the lungs are in disorder.   The vessels are

2. Wang Ping adds: "When the kidneys do not flourish then the marrow is not complete; when the marrow is not complete then the muscles dry up and shrink, hence the joints become bent (have spasms, cramps)."

3. Wang Ping says: " 苛, 'afflictions,' means severe numbness(痹重)."

4. Wang Ping says: "The stomach is the ocean for the nourishment."

not in harmony with the main vessels which ascend and descend. Hence the main vessels are restrained and cannot function, and man suffers from a disease of the veins.[5]

"If, however, the habits of life are as usual and breathing is noisy; and if one cannot rest, or if one rests there is troubled breathing, then something has temporary residence in the breath; water follows the saliva and moves. The water of the kidneys influences the saliva, disturbs the rest, and causes the troubled breathing."

The Emperor said: "Excellent!"

5. "The *Nei Ching* employs three different characters to designate vessels. Their meaning and function are never very exactly described. "The terms *chin* [ching] 經, *loh* 絡, and *sun* 孫 are employed to designate the type of vessels. Broadly speaking they correspond to the arteries, veins, and capillaries. But this distinction is not often clearly made." See Wong and Wu, *History of Chinese Medicine*, loc. cit. p. 19.

INDEX

Acupuncture, 2, 8, 53, 56–78, 83, 107, 111, 118, 123, 143, 146–150, 152, 157, 186, 187, 192–204, 209–211, 213, 215–219, 221–226, 228, 231, 243–246, 249

Aging, 17, 20, 97–100, 121, 182, 183

Air, 49–51, 62, 70, 116–248 passim

Alarm. See Emotions

Albright, William F., 6

Albuminoids, 65, 74

Amenorrhea, 128, 250

Anatomy, 2–4, 6, 25, 30, 49

Anesthesia, 3

Anger. See Emotions

Angina pectoris, 165

Angiology, 50

Animals, 55, 112–206 passim

Anus. See Orifices

Anxiety. See Emotions

An-yang, 6

Armor, 5

Artemisia vulgaris, 65

Arteries. See Vessels

Astrology, 97

Astronomy, 21, 101–223 passim

Atmospheric influence, 11, 14, 18, 21, 23, 24, 34, 42, 47, 49–51, 56, 65, 68, 72, 98–251 passim

Atom bomb, 75

Ayurvedic medicine, vi

Back, 51, 110–249 passim

Baths, 180

Bertholet, A., 11

Bladder, 17, 21, 30, 34, 37, 62, 100–245 passim

Bleeding, 130, 189, 204, 205, 210

Blindness. See Vision, impairment of

Blood, 24, 34, 50, 51, 53, 55, 62, 65, 68, 70, 74, 75, 99–252 passim

Blood vessels. See Vessels

Bodde, Derk, 97

Bones, 21, 23, 24, 30, 50, 54, 55, 62, 99–252 passim

Bowels, 25, 28, 30, 48, 49, 53, 58, 100–240 passim

Brain, 30, 145

Breath; breathing, 34, 45, 47, 50, 53, 55, 56, 62, 68, 81, 88, 101–253 passim

Buddhism, 10, 11, 72, 73, 75

Castration, 3

Celestial stems, 24, 42, 135–246 passim

Chalcolithic, 6

Chalmers, P., 13

Chang Chi. See Chang Chung-ching

Chang Chung-ching, 8, 77, 78, 84, 88

Chang-sha, 8, 77

Chang Shih-hsien, 44

Chang (Tao)-ling, 82

Chao Ming Yin Chih, 85

Chavannes, Édouard, 5, 97

Ch'ên Hsiu-yüan, 26

Chest, 51, 75, 110–247 passim

Chi, 5

Chi Tzu, 89

Ch'i lin, 5

Ch'i Pai, 6

Chia Yu, 89

Ch'ia I-ching, 8, 77, 88

Chien Lung, 77

Chills, 51, 102–251 passim

Chin, 52

Ch'in dynasty, 8, 18, 77, 88

Ch'in Ho, 88

Ch'in Yüeh-jên. See Pien Ch'iao

Ch'ing dynasty, 26

Chou, duke of, 89

Chou dynasty, 6, 82, 88, 89

Chronomancy, 97

Chung Yung, 7, 213

Ch'un Ch'iu, 88

Ch'un Yu-i, 3, 82
Ch'üan Yüan-ch'i, 77, 78, 88
Climatic conditions. *See* Atmospheric influence
Clothes, 85, 98–252 *passim*
Coix Lachryma, 183
Colors, 21, 42, 47, 50, 52, 85, 112–246 *passim*
Compass, points of the, 20, 21, 24, 34, 42, 55, 105–147 *passim*
Complexion, 52, 54, 57, 149–246 *passim*
Conception, 130
Confucianism, 3, 4, 7, 10, 11, 18, 88
Confucius, 3, 10, 11, 18, 88
Constipation, 111, 121, 182
Cosmogony. *See* Creation
Cough, 24, 47, 50, 83, 109–250 *passim*
Cowdry, E. V., 4
Creation, 10, 13–15, 19, 22, 30, 34, 42, 54, 58, 62, 70, 74, 104, 115, 118–120, 147
Cure. *See* Treatment

Dabry, P., 59, 66, 67
Dawson, Percy M., 7
Deafness. *See* Hearing, impairment of
Death, 14, 15, 17, 45, 47, 51, 54, 82, 87, 105–252 *passim*
Deformity, 107, 161
Diagnosis, 3, 16, 42, 43, 45, 47, 49, 54, 57, 75, 106–253 *passim*
Diaphragm, 45, 51, 165–248 *passim*
Diarrhoea, 103, 110, 129
Diet, 50, 54, 56, 97, 98, 123, 138, 145–148, 150, 151, 156, 159, 180, 186, 195, 200–203, 205–207, 233, 237
Digestion, 30, 100
Disease, 2, 14, 16, 17, 24, 42, 43, 47–58, 65, 70, 72, 74–76, 78, 102–253 *passim*
Dissection, 25
Dreams, 47, 163
Dropsy, 115, 156, 165, 181, 185

Drugs. *See* Medicines
Dualism, 11–15, 65
Dubs, Homer H., 4, 8
Ducts. *See* Vessels
Du Halde, J. P., 1

Ears, 21, 22, 51, 105–242 *passim*
East India Companies, 1, 73
Eckstein, Oskar, 2
Elements, 10, 13, 16, 18–23, 30, 34, 42, 50, 54, 78, 89, 104–251 *passim*
Elimination, 25, 28, 50, 100
Emory College, 75
Emotions, 21, 28, 42, 50, 87, 101–232 *passim*
Environment, 55, 56, 72, 147–149, 195
Erh Ya, 187
Ethics, 10, 12
Etiology, 12, 16, 17, 23, 24, 42, 43, 45, 47, 49, 50–55, 65, 70, 72, 78, 82, 98–252 *passim*
Examination, 42, 43, 47, 53, 113–226 *passim*
Extremities, 34, 45, 56, 60, 61, 110–252 *passim*
Eyes, 21, 22, 34, 42, 51, 105–250 *passim*

Fan Ching-jen, 6
Fear. *See* Emotions
Feet, 34, 52, 62, 122–252 *passim*
Fevers, 30, 50–52, 56, 75, 109–250 *passim*; intermittent, 24, 52, 102, 109–111
Fitzgerald, C. P., 5, 6
Five Canons, 10, 17, 22
Flavors, 21, 23, 34, 42, 54–56, 87, 89, 109–213 *passim*
Flesh, 23, 34, 50, 51, 54, 99–252 *passim*
Foci, the Three. *See* Spaces, The Three Burning
Food. *See* Diet
Forke, Alfred, 13, 14, 19, 22, 87
Four Books, 7
Franke, Otto, 11, 13, 14, 18

Fruit, 55, 205, 206
Fu-hsi, 81, 89
Fu Pao, 5
Fu Sang, 83
Fujikawa, Y., 73
Fung Yu-lan, 97

Gall Bladder, 16, 21, 28, 31, 51, 59, 100–243 *passim*
Generation, gestation, 28
Genitals, 213, 240, 241
Giles, Herbert Allen, 5, 79, 89
Giraffe, 5
Grain, 21, 55, 112–248 *passim*
Groot, J. J. M. de, 12, 17, 25, 87, 97
Growth, 20, 21, 28, 98, 99, 102
Grube, Wilhelm, 11, 97

Hackmann, Erich, 11, 13, 20
Hair, 20, 21, 24, 98–180 *passim*
Han dynasty, 6, 8, 9, 48, 77, 81, 83, 90
Han Shu, 77
Hands, 34, 43–46, 48, 52, 62, 122–249 *passim*
Hauer, Erich, 3
Head, 28, 51, 106–249 *passim*
Headache, 143–243 *passim*
Health, 14, 17, 42, 47, 58, 75, 76, 104–221 *passim*
Hearing, 108, 115, 122, 152; impairment of, 51, 101, 109, 122, 158, 204, 233, 240, 246
Heart, 16, 20, 22–25, 28, 30, 34, 36, 43, 45, 47, 50, 52, 59, 63, 88, 100–250 *passim*
Heaven, 11–15, 18, 19, 42, 53, 82, 85, 87, 97–235 *passim*
Hemiplegia, 232
Hemoglobin, 74
Hernia, 129, 144, 180
Hersey, John, 75
Hiroshima, 75
Hollow Spaces. *See* Bowels
Hon-Han-shu, 3, 82
Honan, 6
Hospitals, 1

Hsiao Erh T'ui Na Kuang I, 46
Hsieh, E. T., 6, 25, 28, 59, 62
Hsien-yüan, 5
Hsin-Chia Ching, 111
Hsüan Chu, 85
Hsüeh Chi, 78
Huang-fu Mi, 8, 77, 88
Huang-ti, 4, 81
Hua T'o, 3, 8, 82
Hübotter, Franz, 3, 28, 240
Huizenga, Lee S., 4
Hume, Edward H., 2, 3, 10
Hunan, 77

I Ching, 10, 15, 79
I Tsung Pi Tu, 41
I Yin, 89
Illness. *See* Disease
Impotence, 20, 98–232 *passim*
Injury. *See* Disease
Insanity. *See* Mental disturbance
Insects, 163
Intercourse, sexual. *See* Relations, sexual
Intestines, 16, 17, 21, 28, 30, 32, 33, 38, 45, 59, 62, 64, 100–243 *passim*

Japan, 2, 69–76, 83
Jaundice, 172
Jên Tsung, 89
Jesuits, 1
Job's Tears. *See* Coix Lachryma
Joints, 34, 62, 105–252 *passim*
Joy. *See* Emotions

Kaempfer, Engelbert, 69, 71
Kang-Hsi, 48, 217
Kao Pao-hêng, 9, 85, 90
Kidneys, 17, 21, 26, 28, 30, 36, 38, 43, 45, 47, 49, 52, 62, 63, 98–253 *passim*
K'ung An-kuo, 81

Lancing, 211, 213, 214, 231, 232
Lao-tzu, 7, 10, 11, 189
Latourette, K. S., 1
Lee T'ao, 4

Legge, James, 81
Legs. *See* Extremities
Lei Kung, 87
Leprosy, 49
Leucocytes, 74, 75
Lieh-tze, 13
Ligaments, 21, 59, 62
Liki, 22
Limbs. *See* Extremities
Lin I, 9, 78, 79, 85, 90
Ling Shên, 138
Ling Shu Su Wên Cheh Yao Ch'ien Chu, 26, 27, 29, 31–33, 35–40, 63, 64, 81
Littré, Émile, 72
Liu Shao, 79
Liver, 10, 21–25, 28–30, 34, 36, 42, 43, 45, 47, 52, 54, 59, 100–245 *passim*
Lockhart, W., 1, 25
Longevity, 12, 17, 18, 50, 81, 85, 90, 97, 98, 100–102, 106, 109, 121
Lü Tsu, 4
Lun Yü, 7
Lungs, 17, 21–25, 28, 34, 36, 43, 45, 47, 50, 52, 62, 100–252 *passim*

Madness. *See* Mental disturbance
Ma-fei-san, 3
Malaria. *See* Fevers, intermittent
Malpractice, 57, 150, 160, 226, 227
Marrow, 24, 30, 54, 108–252 *passim*
Massage, 57, 148, 210, 211, 224
Materia medica. *See* Medicines
Matthews, R. H., 5, 138
Ma-yao, 3
Meat. *See* Animals
Medicine: native, 1, 2, 4, 6, 7, 70, 72, 73; scientific, Western, 1, 2, 4, 6, 49, 57, 73, 74
Medicines, 3, 54–57, 70, 105, 147, 148, 150–152, 154, 180, 181, 206, 210, 211, 231, 249
Meh-Ching, 42, 78
Mencius, 7
Meng-tzu, 7
Menstruation, 20, 98–250 *passim*

Mental disturbance, 49–51, 54, 108–248 *passim*
Metabolism, 74
Mi Huang-fu, 8, 77
Mind, 98, 101–103, 109, 123, 151, 157, 216
Ming dynasty, 9, 44, 78
Mirror, The Golden, 60, 61
Missionary Society of China, Medical, 1
Monad, 13
Morse, H. B., 1
Morse, William R., 25, 28, 53, 59, 70
Mouth, 21, 22, 105–250 *passim*
Moxa, moxibustion, 8, 57–77, 148, 151, 100, 101, 110, 110
Muscles, 20, 21, 23, 24, 30, 42, 54–56, 59, 62, 99–252 *passim*

Nakajama, T., 2, 3, 59, 72–75
Nan Ching, 3, 9, 88, 99, 109, 247
Neck, 47, 50, 51, 109–247 *passim*
Needles. *See* Acupuncture
Nervous disease. *See* Mental disturbance
Nose, 21, 22, 51, 52, 105–245 *passim*
Numbers, system of, 10, 18–21, 30, 34, 38, 43, 49, 50, 52–57, 62, 83, 88, 89, 100–251 *passim*
Numbness, 34, 50, 56, 142–252 *passim*
Nutrition. *See* Diet

Odors, 21, 112–206 *passim*
Opium, 3
Orifices, 21, 22, 30, 58, 61, 105–233 *passim*

Pa Kua, 81, 89
Pain, 3, 50–52, 117–246 *passim*
Palpation, 42–48, 50, 52, 78, 113, 124, 125, 159, 163, 191, 203
Pan Ku, 81
Pao Ying, 75, 85, 88
Paralysis, 49, 56, 106–249 *passim*
Paré, Ambroise, 73
Parenthood, 15, 115

Parturition, 20, 98
Passions. *See* Emotions
Pathology, 42, 43
Peking Union Medical College, 4, 6
Pên Tsao, 81
Pentatonic Scale, 22, 162
Pericardium, 35
Perspiration, 22, 30, 51, 52, 103–250
  passim
Philology, 49, 82
Philosophy, 9–12, 81
Phoenix, 5
Physicians, orthodox Chinese. *See*
  Medicine, native
Physiology, 7, 25, 28, 30, 49
Pien Ch'iao, 3, 82, 88
Pottery, 5, 6
Practitioners, indigenous. *See*
  Medicine, native
Pregnancy, 98, 130, 172
Prevention, 47, 49, 53, 57, 105, 152,
  220
Priorism, 9, 17, 18
Procreativeness, 12, 20, 98–232
  passim
Prognosis, 47, 51, 53, 55, 102–252
  passim
Psychiatry, 151, 156, 157, 203
Pulse, 23, 24, 30, 34, 42–48, 50, 51,
  54, 57, 58, 70, 73, 75, 78, 99–252
  passim

Read, Bernard E., 70
Rectum. *See* Orifices
Regimen, 10, 53, 56, 58, 97–253
  passim
Relations, sexual, 98, 99, 108, 116
Religion, 2–4, 10–12, 53, 73
Respiration. *See* Breath
Rudd, Herbert F., 11

Sages, ancient, 12, 18, 53, 81, 85, 87,
  89, 98–152 *passim*
Sang Yueh, 18
Saussure, Chantepie de la, 11
Seasons, 12, 14, 18–21, 23–25, 30, 43,
  50, 52, 54, 68, 101–235 *passim*

Se-ma Ts'ien. *See* Ssu-ma Ch'ien
Semen, 20, 99, 100, 126
Sexes, 14, 15, 20, 43, 98–100, 145,
  154
Shang dynasty, 6, 89
Shên-nung, 81
Shên Tsung, 8
Shi chi, 3
Shih Ching, 10
Shih Huang-ti, 83
Ships, 5
Shu Ching, 10
Shun, 89
Sickness. *See* Disease
Skin, 21, 23, 24, 62, 65, 74, 83, 85,
  103–239 *passim*
Smells. *See* Odors
Societas Jesu. *See* Jesuits
Soubeiran, J. Léon, 59, 66
Soulié de Morant, G., 2, 59, 72, 73
Spaces, The Three Burning, 27, 28,
  30, 62, 100, 104, 111, 145, 206
Speech. *See* Voice
Splanchnology, 59
Spleen, 16, 21–25, 28, 34, 36, 40, 43,
  45, 50, 52, 59, 109–250 *passim*
Ssu-k'u Ch'üan-shu tsung-mu t'i yao,
  7
Ssu-ma Ch'ien, 3, 5, 97
Ssu-ma Kuang, 6
Stomach, 16, 21, 28, 30, 38, 39, 45,
  52, 62, 64, 99–252 *passim*
Sui dynasty, 8, 77, 83, 88
Sung dynasty, 8, 78, 79, 89, 90
Supernatural, 42
Surgery, 2–4, 58, 153
Swellings, 52, 99–250 *passim*
Symptomatology, 22, 30, 34, 47, 49–
  52, 78, 106–253 *passim*

Ta Hsüeh, 7
T'ai Shan, 83
T'ai Su, 88
Tai T'ing-huai, 22
T'ai Yo. *See* T'ai Shan
T'ang dynasty, 8, 72, 78, 79, 85, 88–
  90

T'ang Ming-huang, 4

Tao, 10–12, 17, 18, 34, 49, 50, 53, 83, 85, 97, 98, 100–102, 104, 105, 109, 113, 118, 121, 133, 134, 153, 154, 178, 186, 215

Taoism, 4, 10–12, 82, 88, 97

Tastes, 112–206 passim

Teeth, 20, 98–247 passim

Terror. See Emotions

Testicles, 20, 99–242 passim

Thorax, 28, 45, 47, 50, 51, 70, 110–250 passim

Throat, 47, 109–235 passim

T'ien Yüan Yü Ts'e, 85

Tokyo, University of, 73

Treatment, 16, 53–76, 115–249 passim

Tsang Kung, 8

Tso Ch'iu-ming, 88

Tso Chuan, 81, 88

Tu fu, 79

T'u Chu Mo-Chüeh, 44

Typhoid fever, 51; Treatise on, 8, 51, 77, 78, 88

Ulcers, 51, 58, 107–133 passim

Unicorn, 5

United States, 4

Universalism, 10, 11, 13, 15, 20, 53, 62, 73, 76, 81, 97

Urethra. See Orifices

Urine, 52, 167, 177, 206, 207, 242, 249, 250

Vegetables, 55, 205

Vessels, 20, 21, 30, 34, 43, 51, 59–65, 83, 99–253 passim

Viscera, 21–25, 28, 30, 38, 41–43, 45, 47, 48, 50, 51, 53, 54, 58, 59, 70, 83, 100–252 passim

Vision, 34, 108–246 passim; impairment of, 106–108, 121, 122, 157, 246

Voice, 42, 50, 52, 109–249 passim; impairment of, 164, 175, 177

Wang Chi-min, 4, 7, 8

Wang Ping, 8, 9, 43, 54, 56, 78, 79, 81, 83, 85, 88, 97, 98, 104–106, 108, 119, 122, 125, 128, 130, 135–138, 140, 142, 145, 146, 150, 154, 160, 161, 163–166, 170, 172, 174, 177, 179–183, 185–192, 195–197, 199–201, 203–205, 207–210, 213, 214, 216, 218–223, 225–236, 239–246, 248–250, 252

Wang Shu-ho, 42

Wang Sien-chien, 81

Way, The, Way, The Right. See Tao

Weather. See Atmospheric influence

Wei dynasty, 82

Wên Wang, 89

Wieger, Léon, 7, 8, 13

Williams, Edward I., 5

Womb, 145

Wong, K. Chimin, 3, 4, 6–8, 18, 45, 59, 87, 143, 252

Wu, Lien-teh, 3, 4, 6, 8, 18, 42, 45, 59, 87, 143, 252

Wylie, Arthur, 7, 10, 79

Yang, 10, 12–17, 19, 22, 25, 30, 34, 42, 43, 47, 50, 58, 59, 62, 65, 68, 70, 74, 75, 78, 82, 87, 97–252 passim

Yang Shang-shan, 88

Yao, 89

Yên Wu-chih, 79

Yin, 10, 12, 13, 15–17, 19, 22, 25, 30, 34, 42, 43, 47, 50, 59, 62, 65, 68, 70, 74, 75, 78, 82, 87, 97–252 passim

Yin dynasty, 6, 89

Yuan Ch'eng-tsung, 4

Yü dynasty, 89, 105

Yu-hsiung, 5

Yung Jung, 7, 77

Zodiac, 85, 223